WHERE MEDICINE FAILS

WHERE

MEDICINE

FAILS

by

Carol E. McMahon, Ph.D.

Previously Published by,
TRADO-MEDIC BOOKS
A Division of Conch Magazine Ltd., Publishers
Owerri   New York   London
1986

First published 1986 by Trado-Medic Books

Printed in the United States of America

Booksurge
7290 B Investment Drive
North Charleston, SC 29418
1-866-308-6235 ext. 6
www.booksurge.com

Library of Congress Cataloging in Publication Data

McMahon, Carol E., 1946-
  Where medicine fails.

  Includes bibliographies.
  1. Medicine, Psychosomatic – Philosophy.   2. Medicine –
Philsophy.   3. Mind and body.   4. Dualism.   5. Holistic
medicine.   I. Title.   [DNLM: 1. Biofeedback (Psychology).
2. Holistic Health.   3. Metaphysics.   4. Philosophy,
Medical.   5. Psychophysiologic Disorders – psychology.
W 61 M478w]
RC49.M37   1986   615.8'51   86-7840
ISBN 1-4392-4193-7
EAN13 978-1-4392-4193-6

To
RNP and MMP

Chapter Outline

Preface

On the occasion of our first meeting a young man sat in my office in a condition of evident discomfort. For several years he had been the victim of severe and often incapacitating headaches. In anxious tones he spoke of numerous and elaborate medical tests he had undergone, all of which failed to disclose a physical basis of symptoms. No form of organic disease, no evidence of physical pathology had been identified, and he said he had rather they "found a brain tumor" than to continue to "live with this."

It was not the pain, however, to which he referred as unendurable. Living with uncertainty as to its cause had proven equally hard to bear and increasingly frustrating. Contrary to his every expectation, medical science had proclaimed him fundamentally healthy, and he had been assured that there was "nothing physically wrong." The word "psychosomatic" had been applied to his complaint, and he had been advised to "learn how to relax."

Thus he appeared in my office prepared to undertake a program of 'self-regulation' training. Biofeedback and other procedures would be employed to assist him in establishing and maintaining a profound state of bodily and mental relaxation. Though he avowed a willingness to comply with instructions, he seemed from various indications to labor under misgivings concerning the probability of successful outcome.

As if by instinct he had resisted the "psychosomatic" classification, finding it satisfactory neither as an explanation of his illness, nor as imparting hopeful prospects for remediation. Indeed, he interpreted "psychosomatic" as more an accusation than a diagnosis. The word seemed to imply that the disease existed primarily "in his mind." Such a disorder was somehow less legitimate or respectable than a condition with a physical cause, and the psychosomatic diagnosis bode ill of the likelihood of a cure.

Rather than representing an isolated instance, this case of headache characterizes a familiar theme and manifests a perennial problem of traditional medicine. The psychosomatic diagnosis embodies a paradox. It implies that the illness is by some means self-inflicted, yet it does not imply what might logically follow, namely, that it should be as easily self-remedied. "Psychosomatic" signifies that "the mind" has been involved in creating the disturbance, yet medical science has no confidence in mind as capable of readjusting functions toward normal, nor any popularly sanctioned therapeutic program to effect such a reversal of the process. We accept, although with justified reluctance, that psychological influences can produce bodily disturbances, and there we stop. In some cases we offer sufferers as little hope as might be derived from the advice to "learn to live with it."

As the chapters of this book explain, this problem of conceiving causes and cures of psychosomatic or "stress related" illnesses is an area in which medicine fails. Yet the conceptual difficulty is not restricted to the medical establishment. The problem resides equally in deep seated convictions harbored by each of us. Throughout our lives we carry a prejudice in the form of a tacit assumption that our bodies are beyond our control. Our minds or egos, our very selves, are but witnesses to the corruption of matter known as disease. For reasons explained herein, this conviction, though little more than an illusion, has had dramatic consequences to the detriment of health and health care.

To compound difficulties, the prejudice inveighs against use of effective methods available today. Self-regulation strategies such as autogenic training, progressive muscle relaxation and procedures known as "standard relaxation exercises," have been well researched and amply documented as reliable, effective and free of adverse side effects. But physicians who might avail themselves of these resources, and even clients in the course training, are often defeated by the prejudice that the human body is beyond the realm of voluntary control. The bias is at times voiced explicitly by the medical establishment, but the lay person typically harbors it implicitly, and it is carried even into the self-regulation training setting. The ironical outcome presents a situation in which one undertakes instruction in performing feats one knows oneself incapable of performing at the outset.

Each of us has a decided preference for illnesses with physical causes to which physical or chemical remedies might be made to apply. In instances where no physical basis of symptoms is apparent, our prejudice can interfere with successful utilization of innovative, holistic methods. After all, who would seriously consider the possibility that one could willfully reduce the secretion of stomach acids thereby reversing the ulcer process? How absurd it would appear that one could master control of blood pressure or acquire ability to regulate the aberrant beating of one's heart. Each of us knows before the fact how negligible the likelihood of eliminating low back pain by establishing command over the very nerves and muscles responsible for the problem, and the prospect of learned control of blood sugar and cholesterol levels seems perfectly absurd. These convictions are as deep seated as any other preconceptions we harbor, and the prejudice they evince is a prejudice against ourselves.

This book identifies the source of this prejudice, and more importantly, shows it to be unfounded. A message of hope is conveyed in the fact that a realization of past errors points our way to their correction. The elimination of old biases permits a revolutionary perspective on health care and health maintenance. It is hoped that the reader may come away from this book with a new perspective on human nature. If this is not the outcome, at least the reader will achieve an awareness of the error in the traditional perception.

For three centuries medical theory and practice have been founded upon a conception of human nature strictly prohibitive of progress in one area. In all cases where the disease process involves "the whole," that is, where physical factors alone cannot furnish complete explanations, in all of these cases traditional medicine fails. The barrier to progress here is so monumental, and so painful to confront, that orthodox medicine has long denied the existence of any problem. As these chapters show, however, no longer we can ignore or deny this embarrassment to modern science. The "whole" of human nature must no longer be concealed. We must go to the very foundations, to the most fundamental underlying principles, and there uproot the prejudice, the error which has blinded us for the past three centuries.

The present treatment is intentionally unencumbered by citations and footnotes characteristic of academic literature. It is my hope that the brief, informal treatment used here will make important concepts accessible to general readers and to time-pressured professionals for whom extensive detail would be burdensome. Readers seeking full documentation are referred to the titles listed as References, to my works in the periodical literature and to my forthcoming title: *The Rise and Fall of Holism: A Critical Analysis of Medicine.*

The research leading to this project could not have been completed had it not been for support from two sources. The American Philosophical Society made possible a period of research at our nation's Library of Congress and National Library of Medicine. The National Institute of Mental Health made possible a period of research abroad where the resources of the Wellcome Institute for the History of Medicine in London proved invaluable.

The project was favorably influenced by the critical scrutiny of Dr. Bruce Rideout of Ursinus College. Drs. M. L. McMahon and R. N. Parikh contributed similar assistance. Margaret Sweet and Mary Gattie Ziewers typed the manuscript. Finally, my indebtedness to my husband and daughter is boundless for their tolerance and strong support throughout.

Carol E. McMahon
Colden, New York
August, 1985

I

Introduction

Only he who knows the innermost nature of man can cure him in
earnest.

Paracelsus (1493-1541)

This book bears witness to the approaching end of an era in modern
medical history. It has become apparent that a fault residing in the
foundation upon which physical medicine rests must invariably lead to
a collapse of existing assumptions regarding the nature of the disease
process.

The fault to which I refer does not lie where one might at first be inclined to direct critical attention. It cannot be identified with the actual
practice of medicine. It is not to be found in specific shortcomings of
existing theory, nor in the areas of diagnosis or therapy. Though
modern medicine has been subject to frequent criticism as overly
mechanistic or physicalistic and therefore dehumanizing, neither can
the tragic flaw be isolated here.

The fault destined to precipitate a conceptual revolution lies instead
at the foundation upon which all else is built, in a hard-core of assumptions concerning the essence of human nature. Medical theory and
practice are governed by a philosophy or "metaphysic" which is tacitly
assumed, seldom articulated, and never brought into question. Known
to philosophers as "mind-body dualism," this metaphysic has determined the course of medical history for the past three centuries.

For every science there exists a metaphysical hard-core of principles
which decide for the practitioner what can and what cannot be considered true. For this reason, a physicist would be unlikely to entertain
the idea that "psychic powers" could disrupt the motion of molecules in
a solution. Such an event fits uncomfortably with the physicist's picture
of the real world. Similarly, we would be unable to persuade a neuro-
scientist that mental entities such as ideas, desires and memories, are
the immediate causes of the firings of nerve cells in the brain. And by
virtue of the same underlying assumptions regarding the real world,
we would find it difficult to convince a physician that by means of "will
power" an individual could voluntarily alter blood chemistry. Body, it

is assumed, is governed exclusively by laws pertaining to matter, and matter is uninfluenced by mind.

Each of these proposals is rejected *a priori* and automatically by scientists. Such ideas seem preposterous because the modern world-picture forbids any interaction between mental and physical dimensions of existence. These proposals violate expectations and set scientists ill at ease. Those who entertain proposals like these step outside the realm of "hard science." They may be called "para-psychologists" from the root "para," meaning "outside of" psychology, but more typically their endeavors are placed in the category of "pseudoscience," meaning no science at all.

Although the underlying metaphysic determines with precision what may be considered true; what may be suitable subjects for inquiry, and what methods a researcher may employ, the metaphysic itself is never brought into question. Science never challenges its philosophic ground plan except in the extraordinary event of "scientific revolution." In this rare instance, so eloquently elucidated in recent years by the philosopher of science, Thomas S. Kuhn, science calls into question its very definition of reality.

In the event of scientific revolutions, world-pictures turn topsy-turvy. Such occurrences have taken humanity from a flat earth at the very center of the cosmos to a small planet revolving around one of a myriad of stars. Three centuries ago a dramatic conceptual upheaval of this type took us from a holistic concept of human nature to our modern perspective of mind-body dualism.

Within the present century a gradual accumulation of knowledge (which includes a realization of the inadequacy of the existing model), has furnished the necessary conditions for another scientific revolution. This body of knowledge must invariably precipitate a conceptual revolution in medicine, one which will restore holism where duality has for three centuries claimed ultimate authority.

The impending revolution to which this book directs attention is not to be mistaken for the modern evolution of concepts of health and health maintenance. The revolution in question cannot be equated with the life-style changes so manifest in our society today. It is not evinced in the vogue of aerobic exercise and the consciousness of good nutrition. It cannot be identified with the avoidance of "stress" as seen in the recent tendency of business executives to refuse to uproot families and change locations for higher salaries. Nor can the revolution be equated with the growing popularity of innovative healing strategies such as biofeedback and other methods of instating "self-regulation."

These are signs of the times. Some reflect unrest and disquietude with traditional, physicalistic medicine, but the revolution to which this book is directed transcends all such vogues and attitude changes. These contemporary modifications of behavior are deviations from the traditional course but they are not outcomes of a conceptual restructuring of medicine. The inevitable revolution will strike the roots of tradition and define human nature anew. It will prove vastly more fundamental and encompassing than all such behavior and attitude changes combined.

The name "holism" has been given to the movement from which many current innovations spring. The movement is not part of medicine proper but moves forward independently and in some instances against the grain of orthodox medical opinion. Practitioners of "holistic healing" are likely to have had no medical training, and from within the medical establishment, formal and informal denouncements of holistic methods are fairly typical responses to innovation.

One might well ask how the health care revolution known as holism can proceed in independence of medicine and why this should be the case. This book answers these questions by demonstrating that "holism" is itself incompatible with traditional scientific medicine. Medical theory rests upon a solid dualistic foundation. Only through the conceptual upheaval for which the stage is now set will the doors of medical science be opened to concepts of the whole.

Dualism and Modern Medical Miracles

Problems regarding lack of holistic understanding of the disease process are seldom voiced by orthodox practitioners. Adherents to an established conceptual model have confidence in its potential to explain all it is necessary or desirable to explain. Difficulties springing from mind-body dualism have remained largely unseen, and when seen, have been minimized in importance.

Media releases from official sources frame announcements in terms of scientific medicine's "triumphs" and "conquests." If total victory cannot be claimed, medicine often proclaims a partial victory with the remainder just around the corner. The smallpox vaccine has wiped the disease from the face of the earth and the AIDS virus has been isolated. When the virus was conclusively identified and produced in large quantities, the Secretary of Health announced: "Today we add another miracle to the long honor roll of American medicine and science." "Miracles of modern technology" have given us greatly publicized organ transplants. Artificial organs are to every indication the wave of the future, and medicine is "within an inch" of a cure of several devastating diseases.

Each of these medical marvels has a common attribute. In every case of conquest or near conquest there exists a "physical cause" of pathology and a physical or physico-chemical remedy. The common factor missing from these diseases and from their remedies is the mental dimension of human existence. Research leading to these triumphs is conducted with the absolute exclusion of mind from realm of causation. Most of what is known today of human disease has come from experiments on animals where no psychological factors have been included in research designs. The challenges which physical medicine masters so well are invariably those uncomplicated by the "whole" of human nature. If the challenge involves a virus or germ, a surgically correctable problem or a chemically induced disturbance, medicine approaches the problem with well founded confidence.

It requires but a superficial glance at medical theory and practice to perceive the underlying assumption that *all* physical diseases do in fact have physical causes. Such has been the historic definition of "real," as opposed to "imaginary" diseases. As we shall see in the following chapter, however, our knowledge of the so-called "stress diseases" has brought physical medicine to an impasse. These disorders stubbornly point to another order of complexity in disease causation, to causes which medical science has been unable to isolate in the research laboratory.

When the disease process refuses to submit to conventional analysis in terms of physico-chemical or mechanistic concepts, scientific medicine stumbles and falls. Where physical explanation reaches its limits without explaining all, the scientist becomes helpless. It is evident today that the key to enlightenment does not lie along the path of progressive expansion of existing research programs. Since medical knowledge is constrained by a dualistic definition of human nature, medical science cannot possibly accommmodate conditions which are incomprehensible apart from the whole. The so-called "stress diseases" refuse to submit to conventional analysis in terms of mechanistic causation.

Were it not for dualism, however, we would never have benefited from the triumphs of physical medicine. Had the body never been conceived as an uncomplicated physico-chemical mechanism, medicine should never have been prompted to mechanistic solutions like artificial hearts, pacemakers and implants. Medicine's triumphs have indeed been as mighty as those of the kindred physical sciences, chemistry, physics, and engineering. The magnitude of its victories has helped to sustain the illusion that all disease was ultimately within the reach of physical medicine.

1. Traditional Medicine and the Unseen Whole

Around the turn of the nineteenth century a physician wrote the epigram: "It is much more important to know what sort of person has a disease than what sort of disease he has." Thought provoking little gems of wisdom like this are found occasionally in medical literature of the past three centuries. Never, however, have such insights been treated as scientific "facts," nor have they formed the basis of medical theories. Principles concerning "persons" are generally agreed to be para-scientific. They force us beyond body and beyond mechanism into an unexplored expanse — the void between matter and mind which for present purposes may be termed "the whole."

As far as science is concerned, all bodily processes have control switches which operate by means of physico-chemical mechanisms. The bodily states of arousal which correspond to emotional experience are triggered by chemical substances known as hormones. Release of adrenalin is triggered by the presence of another hormone, the presence of which is in turn accounted for by physico-chemical brain mechanisms. Science founded upon mind-body dualism forbids entry of non-physical variables into these chains of causation. There are no mental triggers, and no holistic triggers.

Since it would appear utter nonsense to attempt to add non-physical causes to a chain of physical events, science is disinclined to entertain such notions and remains content with the picture as it stands. Because the picture appears complete as is, no problem is visible to the eye of science. There simply is no "whole" inherent in our definition of human nature. Independent and isolated, mind and matter explain all observable phenomena.

Modern science divides all that exists into two categories of entities: those physical and those mental. The former are science's stock in trade, tangible substances, manipulable, observable; atoms and molecules, elements and compounds, and the chemically and physically constituted tissues of the body. All of these can be exhaustively analyzed in terms of the properties of matter. That which is known of these science proudly proclaims to be "hard facts."

The remaining dimension of reality, the mental realm, is definable only by the opposites of the physical world. Events in this category have no shape, size, magnitude or material dimension. They have no substance, no weight, no physical properties whatsoever. They are our ideas, images, memories, emotions and all of the constituents of the stream of consciousness. These are beings 'from another world' which can under no circumstances touch, contact or influence events in the material dimension.

According to scientific medicine, human nature is thus conceived. The mental and physical dimensions of existence entail all that goes into the making of an organism. Our bodies and minds are isolated, separate and fundamentally incompatible. They cannot be added together in such a way as to form a whole which is greater than the sum of its parts.

Scientific medicine occupies itself with the material dimension of human existence. It need not expend energies pondering the essence of "the whole," since no whole exists by definition. For modern medicine "holism" is the name given to a goal, which though somewhat alluring, proves ultimately inaccessible. Neither logical reasoning nor the outcomes of scientific research can form a unity of the mutually exclusive entities − mind and body.

Given our present definition of reality, even the question of what holism might represent is impossible to formulate. In the past, those who have claimed that mental causes operate in disease formation, or that mental cures reverse physical diseases, have been hurriedly and very easily discredited. Rationality is on the side of traditional medicine which permits none other than *physical* causes of physical events.

Medicine, observing itself, sees no problem inherent in its model of human nature. All observations fit nicely into one category or the other. Mind and matter seem to accommodate all events with no surplus remaining and nothing in between. Medicine is thus blind to its central problem. But the eye can be made to see itself if one makes use of a mirror, and we are fortunate in having a mirror by means of which to observe the evolution of the current medical dilemma. The mirror of history reflects our problem with vivid clarity. The present volume makes use of evidence from the past to demonstrate the impediment to progress posed by the philosophic assumption of dualism of mind and body.

Without being able to make a telescopic observation of a celestial body, an astronomer may at times be assured of its existence by numerous other signs — phenomena which would not occur in the absence of its influence. We stand in a similar position today, having accumulated an abundance of evidence for the existence of another dimension of human nature herein referred to as the whole.

Yet the evidence furnished by scientific research findings is never sufficient to precipitate scientific revolution. No amount of criticism of an existing conceptual model, and no proliferation in the number of events it cannot explain, can revolutionize a science when metaphysical roots remain intact. For scientific revolution to occur the metaphysical hard-core of assumptions must be discarded and replaced by an alternative with new defining properties. A philosophic assumption of holism cannot be reconciled with the received view. If holism is to occupy the position of a determinant of medical theory and practice, holism must replace dualism. The mind-matter metaphysic is the source of our difficulties, and that metaphysic itself has been proven untenable.

The Inevitability of Revolution

As previously noted, the stage is at present set for a revolutionary development. The die has been cast. The makings of a conceptual upheaval have sprung from what may appear a surprising source — the science of matter, physics itself. In recent decades several physicists have arrived independently at the same unsettling realization — the laws of physics pertaining to matter are incompatible with the behavior of the matter of living substances such as body tissue. The immaterial mind cannot assume responsibility here by accounting for the behavior of vital matter. Thus it appears that the mind-matter dichotomy as an all-encompassing definition of reality is inadequate.

As the Nobel Prize winning physicist Erwin Schrödinger put it, the behavior of living matter has proven fundamentally different from anything physicists have dealt with in their research laboratories or mentally at their writing desks. Not only do physic's laws pertaining to matter fail to accommodate the phenomena of living tissue, these events seem incompatible with, and contradictory to the rules of physical science.

Though unsettling indeed, this discovery is but one half of the problem physicists have unveiled in recent decades. The other difficulty is similarly related to the philosophic assumption that all reality divides neatly into the categories of mind and matter. It has long been believed that the existence of consciousness did not violate the laws of physics. Brain matter, it was assumed, could by some inexplicable means generate the phenomena described as "mental," without itself being influenced by mental events. For a variety of reasons physicists have been forced to conclude that this model is not workable, and that physical processes are in fact incapable of generating conscious processes. The existence of mind, sentience and intelligence can never be made compatible with the known laws of physics or physical chemistry.

The problem of accounting for consciousness and the impossibility of explaining the phenomena of vital matter point to the same inevitable conclusion regarding a flaw in our world-picture. We are forced to conclude that the division of all existence into mind and matter – the metaphysic known as dualism, is itself at fault. There appears to be but one solution to this problem and that is a revolutionary revision of the world-picture to include a third dimension of reality.

This new realm of existence, which has been called the "biotonic phase," is reducible neither to mental events nor to material events as described by the laws of physics. It has been conceived instead as a totally unique dimension of reality; as a "primary phenomenon." Put in simple terms, this third realm of being encompasses the phenomena which mind and matter cannot accommodate. It includes the properties and functions which accrue to matter in its living form. The metaphysic honored by modern science has mistakenly omitted *life* from the defining principles of the real world. The whole of human nature, unfathomable in the realms of mind and matter, resides in the biotonic dimension.

2. Objectives of the Present Work

The following chapters employ the mirror of history to demonstrate where dualistic medicine fails, as well as the causes of those failures. There was a time when medicine was holistic and approached health and disease in a way dramatically different from the modern approach. The whole of human nature, once clearly apprehended, was lost sight of with the instatement of the dualistic metaphysic which defined the organism in exclusive terms of mind and matter. We will observe how this momentous problem for medicine has been ignored, denied and otherwise circumvented by scientists who have found the truth too painful to confront.

Finally, these chapters point to the biotonic solution, as yet stated only in vague, general terms, awaiting thorough treatment. We are presented with a gaping void, a rift between mind and matter, waiting to be filled with new knowledge concerning the essence of human nature. We have come to a position of certainty that we can no longer conceive human nature in exclusive terms of mind and matter. The new definition, based on an assumption of holism, will give medicine an urgently needed new perspective on the disease process, and will explain a number of events heretofore classified as "medical mysteries."

For three centuries the great hope of physical medicine has been that all illness will be curable when the laws governing matter are fully and precisely elaborated. We find ourselves now, however, in a position of certainty that this expectation has been unfounded. A class of disorders, alternately called "psychosomatic" and "stress diseases," have proven incomprehensible apart from the whole, and medicine has been ill-prepared to handle this category of pathology.

The metaphysic known as dualism has placed medicine on the horns of a dilemma. To explain the 'relationship' between mind and body a choice has been forced between two equally objectionable alternatives: (1) either no relationship exists between mind and body, or (2) mental events exert influences on physical processes and vice versa. In the first instance mind is irrelevant to bodily functions and plays absolutely no role in health or disease. In the second, we assert a causal relationship between mental and physical processes which is logically impossible by definition. This book illustrates how this dilemma has shaped modern medicine and prohibited successful handling or disorders incomprehensible apart from "the whole."

The present work has three primary objectives: (1) to demonstrate the inability of modern medical science to conceptualize or to remedy the so-called "stress disorders" — conditions also known as "psycho-physiologic" or "psychosomatic;" (2) to explain how this failure is a product of our dualistic understanding of human nature; and (3) to demonstrate that dualism is itself untenable. The division of all existence into mind and matter is unacceptable on logical grounds.

It is hoped that a clear understanding of present difficulties will help move us more rapidly toward the new frontier. Its past triumphs notwithstanding, modern medicine faces its greatest challenge today, and a scientific revolution is waiting in the wings.

II

Medicine's Central Problem

> No theoretician has been able to formulate the mind-body relationship in terms which are satisfactory to all. Until this has been done there will always remain a gap which defies attempts to build a unitary theory.
>
> *MacLeod, Wittkower and Margolin, 1954*

1. Disease of the Whole: Remedy of the Parts

a. The "Stress" Diseases

Traditional medicine divides all forms of pathology into two categories: there are "physical" disorders and there are "mental" disorders. This organizational scheme, however, has been thwarted by a class of conditions which betray a third dimension between mind and body, and diseases in this ambiguous area have constituted a thorn in the side of traditional medicine. Over the years they have been subject to several controversial types of interpretation, none of which has achieved lasting official scientific status. The names given to this category of disorders have been: nervous, psychogenic, psychosomatic and stress diseases.

Each historic attempt at explanation, seeking in vain to close the gap between mind and body, has been felled by the established dualistic model. This chapter explains how the concepts employed have failed to capture the true meaning of this class of diseases, since the disorders in question have proven incomprehensible apart from the whole of human nature. They have defeated modern medical science because that science has not yet seen the whole, and remains constrained to frame explanation in dualistic terms.

What do the following conditions have in common?

Low back pain	Diarrhea
Hives	High blood pressure
Constipation	Headache
Ulcers	Indigestion

The reader may suspect a relationship, but should be surprised at how far the relationship extends. In all of their commonalities these disorders represent not merely medical problems, but problems for the science of medicine. The link which ties them resides in the mysterious void between mind and body. Let us survey the interpretations given to these ever present but still unintelligible diseases, and examine the consequences of these interpretations for the sufferer.

Psychosomatic Conditions and Mental Causes of Bodily Disease

In recent years all of these conditions have been grouped under the heading "psychosomatic." "Psyche" refers here to mind and "soma" to body. The word psychosomatic came into use roughly half a century ago when scientists became convinced that diseases of the body could by some unknown mechanism be caused by mental events.

The concept of mental or psychological causation of bodily disturbances was an unsettling revelation for traditional medicine. For centuries that notion had been forbidden on logical grounds. That ideas or emotions could alter physical mechanisms seemed perfectly incredible to scientists. These were events forbidden by logic and by the rules of science. Like "psychokinesis," where mental powers are said to move physical objects, these events were beyond the realm of possibility.

Nevertheless, medicine reluctantly accepted the concept of psychosomatic disease because ample evidence attested to its reality. The evidence was bolstered by a clinical finding which seemed to prove beyond question the involvement of mental factors. It was Dr. Sigmund Freud, the founder of psychoanalysis, who convinced skeptics of the reality of mental causation. He demonstrated that psychotherapy could cure a variety of apparently 'physical' conditions. If a mental remedy could remove a symptom, that symptom must have had a mental cause. Thus Freud argued for "psychogenesis," the creation of bodily disturbances by mental causal factors. The hypothesis of psychogenesis became widely used to explain psychosomatic disease, so widely in fact that early proponents of psychosomatic concepts felt that the new movement would revolutionize medicine.

Let us consider a case in point to demonstrate the operation of this causal principle. Our subject is a young woman whose life has been disrupted by a responsibility imposed upon her — the care of an elderly parent. Her father is gravely ill and requires constant attention. Out of compassion and a sense of duty she forsakes other plans to devote time to his care.

One evening while at his bedside she hears a group of young people passing by outside, laughing and enjoying their carefree existence. Suddenly she feels a tingling sensation in her hand which grows more severe and by the following morning she has developed a complete paralysis of the right arm. She has lost all power of movement in the limb and hand, and she is not pretending or feigning symptoms. The paralysis is real.

Medicine looks to the brain and nerves for an explanation of paralysis, but in this instance, no evidence of organic pathology is found by physical examination. The psychological examination, however, is more revealing and a psychoanalytic investigation reveals a cause. It resides beneath the level of consciousness in a secret and forbidden impulse. While hypnotized the woman discloses a hostile urge to end her father's life, to free her from the burden of his care. The right arm, which might have executed the unthinkable deed, was rendered helpless by the paralysis. Through psychoanalysis she comes to deal consciously with repressed hostilities, and ultimately regains full use of her limb.

This instance of paralysis represents causation by "psychogenesis." Several decades ago, any physical condition successfully treated by psychological intervention was said to represent psychological causation. Many disorders formerly explained in physical or mechanistic causal terms came to be viewed as psychogenic. They included cases of paralysis, blindness, deafness and loss of sensation in the skin, as well as disorders of internal or visceral bodily functions, such as nausea and vomiting, diarrhea, constipation, asthma, fainting or brief loss of consciousness and numerous other common ailments.

In diagnostic manuals and medical reference works a new classification of disease appeared. It was called "psychosomatic" or "psychophysiologic." It involved disorders of the functioning of organs such as heart, stomach and colon, and the causal mechanism of such functional disturbances was said to be psychogenesis.

By the late 1940s the matter appeared settled. Not only were psychological causes real, but in two thirds of his patients the physician was advised to come to grips with the "mechanism" whereby psychological problems find bodily expression.

A vast amount of research on psychosomatic illness, however, failed to elucidate that obscure "causal mechanism," and the logical difficulty of uniting mind and body began to take its toll on the concept of psychogenesis. Science awakened to the harsh reality that no possible mechanism could be conceived whereby mind could influence body. Use of the term psychogenesis waned, and in the present decade it is no longer employed to describe causation of psychosomatic illness.

Medical Mysteries

Thus headaches, low back pain, ulcers and so on were classified as "psychosomatic," and were for a time explained by psychogenesis. Difficulties in obtaining satisfactory causal explanations of these conditions united them through another commonality. When the hypothesis of psychogenesis was found inadequate, these disorders reverted back to the status occupied prior to the influence of Freud. As far as the role of mind was concerned, they became again medical mysteries.

If we disregard psychological influences, however, and hold fast to physical explanations, we dispel the aura of mystery and stand on the firm ground of orthodox scientific medicine. We can say, in the case of headache, for instance, as many still do, that the *physical cause* simply has not yet been identified. We may then proceed in our research with confidence that intensive investigation will ultimately reveal all, and lead to a physico-chemical remedy. We may search for a virus or perhaps a genetic predisposition. We may search for a chemical imbalance, a toxin or nutritional deficiency to label as culprit. If, however, we call mental influences into play, we depart from the firm ground of hard science, and enter into the realm of the mysterious and inexplicable.

"Stress" Diseases

Mental causes of physical diseases are forbidden by logic, yet despite this fact, medicine has been forced to confront the possibility of this enigmatic form of causation. Evidence of apparent mind-body interaction stubbornly and persistently presents itself. In recent years the appearance of self-contradiction has been minimized by evasive tactics in the use of terminology. Rather than affirming psychological causation in explicitly mentalistic language (i.e., "fear caused his arteries to constrict"), science has devised a cunning and effective semantic subterfuge as a means of concealing the underlying mystery. It has borrowed a term from the 'hardest' of hard sciences, physics, and applied that term to explain causation of psychosomatic disease. Thus the concept of "stress-disease" is another factor uniting our psychosomatic conditions, and each of the disorders in question has been causally linked to "stress."

When we look to the origins of the word stress, however, we are surprised to find that "psyche" is by no means a necessary component of the idea. The concept of stress has long been used in physics and engineering to refer to physical forces exerted upon physical objects. In physics, stress is an influence precisely defined, measured and timed. Engineers make use of two associated concepts — stress and strain. "Stress" refers to a force applied to an object, and "strain" describes the effect produced. Stress and strain are measured in terms of force per unit area: kilograms per square centimeter, pounds per square inch, and so on. "Stress" derives from the Latin verb *stringere,* to "draw tight or press together." Thus in the language of science stress is a *physical* variable.

In medicine, however, the term has acquired a diversity of possible meanings, none of which seems evidently preferable to the rest, and thus ambiguity reigns. The vitamin industry has derived considerable benefit from the ambiguity of the stress concept. The word "stress" has been used in the marketing of nutritional supplements. A package label bearing the word carries the clear implication that these tablets reduce or counteract the effects of stress. In all likelihood persons with stress related disorders are consuming these tablets with a misbegotten therapeutic objective.

The medical concept of stress originated in the works of Hans Selye, a distinguished Canadian physiologist, and there was no ambiguity in Selye's *original* use of the word. He dealt exclusively with physical influences on physical processes. Some of the animal subjects in Selye's research were given doses of poison insufficient to kill. Others were exposed to extremes of temperature, or spun round in centrifuges at high speeds. These were physical stresses yet their outcomes on bodily organs were found to resemble the disorders rampant in human beings in our modern era where physical stresses are seldom found.

Selye observed that organisms responded to threatening influences through a series of predictable bodily responses. In their struggle to adapt to stressors Selye's animal subjects showed an initial "alarm reaction." This state of activation prepared the organism for combat. It produced changes which would further ability to fight or to run away and thus to escape the threat.

In this "fight or flight" response circulating blood is redistributed to the muscles used in fighting or running. The heart works harder to ready the organism for vigorous defensive action with an increase in volume of blood pumped with each beat and an increase in blood pressure. As adrenalin pours into the blood stream, the lungs are stimulated to more vigorous respiration. Blood sugar levels rise as stores of glucose are released for quick energy availability.

If these defensive reactions are not terminated by escape from the threat, the animal continues to resist the stressor with continued heightened activation. But this stage of resistance cannot go on indefinitely without depleting the body's resources and creating irreversible damage.

The final stage of the stress reaction observed by Selye was unmistakably similar to the health consequences of human life in the Age of Anxiety. Selye called it "exhaustion." He noted evidence of destruction in the digestive system, in heart and blood vessels, and in the immune system's ability to fight infection. The typical outcome of the stress response in this final stage of exhaustion was death.

From out of this scientific research emerged our modern concept of "stress." Stress is popularly believed to be the cause of each of the disorders listed at the head of this chapter, and more. Current estimates from official sources claim that seventy percent of all illness is due to stress. Yet humans are seldom spun around at high speeds or given sub-lethal does of poison. The actual physical stressors used by Selye to study the phenomenon are almost totally lacking in the environment of humans. We are, in fact, as physically sheltered as one might perhaps desire to be.

The link between stress and ulcers, hypertension and so on, in humans, is a link between mental and bodily events. The cause cannot be accounted for in physical terms. Thus, again, despite widespread use of stress as an explanatory principle, our selection of disorders remains unified by the central problem; an enigma of causation. "Stress" does not diminish, but rather evades the gap between mind and body.

We have found the disorders heading this chapter occupying three categories. They have been called "psychosomatic," they have been causally linked to "stress" and they remain medical mysteries at the most fundamental level of explanation. The problem of explanation leads to a fourth commonality: these disorders have not lent themselves to cures by traditional methods of physical medicine.

Incurable Conditions

The psychosomatic condition has no *physical cause* which can be eliminated by clinical methods used to cure other bodily diseases. There is no germ, for instance, and no virus involved here. There exists no vaccine, and no miracle drug like penicillin to eradicate and prevent recurrence of the stress disorder. Nor is there any organic derangement making possible a cure by surgical procedure, radiation therapy or chemotherapy as used in treatment of cancer.

Stress related disorders are "functional;" they represent disturbances of ongoing processes. They are typically exaggerations of bodily functions which are otherwise normal. High blood pressure, for instance, is perfectly appropriate during the fight or flight defense. If it remains elevated, however, when the threat is no longer present, it is considered a disease. Similarly, muscles are designed to tense and to relax, but a persistence of excessive tension is a functional error which can lead to a variety of psychosomatic complaints such as headache and backache.

A person consulting a physician is likely to have the expectation that a cure will be forthcoming. But the medications prescribed for the stress disorders are not "cures" per se. Rather, they temporarily readjust functioning toward normal. When the medication is discontinued, the functional disturbance typically reappears and in some instances, in an exaggerated degree. Medical opinion links many severe cases of insomnia and constipation to prior use of medications for these conditions. Chemical and surgical treatments fail to cure the stress disorders.

Another commonality among these conditions compounds the problem they represent for public health. Statistics indicate that their occurrence is so frequent that every individual is likely to succumb to one or more of these disorders in the course of a lifetime. This type of pathology, however, does not rage in the less stressful environments of other societies. The epidemic is, in a sense, of our own creation.

A Self-inflicted Epidemic

Stress diseases, whether we wish to admit it or not, are self-inflicted. We do not refer here to malingering, pretending, or desiring to be ill. We refer instead to habits of thought and behavior, accepted as normal by society, which lead to the formation and perpetuation of symptoms of disease.

Stress disease onset is typically gradual. Early warning signals are sounded oftentimes, but to no avail. Were we to detect a lump or hardening in the flesh, or if we observed the presence of blood in urine or feces, we would be moved to take prompt action to identify and eliminate the cause. The early warnings for stress disorders, however, do not prompt immediate action. We accept and live with bouts of diarrhea, excesses of stomach acidity, twitches above the eye and twinges in the lower back. We cultivate ulcers and court coronaries as if bent on determining our own causes of death.

The individual is not entirely to blame in all of this however. Immediate medical attention to a muscle twitch or stomach upset is highly unlikely to bring about the desired result of prevention or cure. Though medicine has a vague notion that persons are producing these disorders by way of stress, it has no method for reversing the process. Medical intervention becomes effective only when warning signals have evolved into observable forms of pathology such as bleeding ulcers, obstructed coronary arteries and structural damage to the back.

Nevertheless, a great deal is known of the self-inflicted character of psychosomatic illness. In the early years of dawning of awareness of mind-body relationships in disease, Dr. Franz Alexander and his colleagues made dramatic progress toward elucidating those relationships. Dr. Alexander was born in Budapest in 1891, and in 1921 received an award from Freud for the best psychoanalytic essay of the year. The psychoanalysts looked for causes in the "unconscious mind." A specific relationship was presumed to exist between physical symptoms and unconscious mental processes. The relationship was meaningful and predictable showing body to be a mirror of mind. In asthma, for instance, Dr. Alexander saw "a suppressed cry for mother." Psychoanalytic investigations found asthmatics to have excessive unresolved dependency on their mothers, and pathology seemed to arise in association with the threat of separation from mother's protection.

Essential hypertension or high blood pressure was found to speak the same meaningful language. Dr. Alexander described its association with hostile impulses and fear of retaliation; with inhibition of those hostile impulses and an ongoing state of anxiety. Such a complex of attributes is analogous to the activation or arousal described by Selye in the context of stress. It reflects the character of the fight or flight response well known to be associated with elevations of blood pressure.

Dr. Alexander's perspective derived from the Freudian model of psychogenesis. But this model failed to furnish the basis for medical theory it seemed at first to promise. The causal link between mental and physical events remained shrouded in mystery and for this reason, concepts of causation gave way to a new method of conceiving the subject matter: correlations. A correlation refers to the simultaneous occurrence of two events. Rather than assert that physical events are *caused by* mental events, science took the safer more conservative route and affirmed that mental and bodily events merely corresponded temporally or occurred together.

Dr. David Graham, a modern leader in psychosomatic medicine, took up the subject matter of psychogenesis and researched it in the modern correlation framework. The mental factors he dealt with were "attitudes." His results revealed the same type of meaningful relationship as had Dr. Alexander's between mental states and physical symptoms. The body seemed a mirror of mind; the two spoke the same words in different languages.

In hypertension, for instance, the attitude found to correlate with the disease was a feeling of having been threatened and having to be "ready for anything." Confirmation of this relationship came from several types of findings. In one case, hypnotized persons to whom the attitude was suggested showed the expected increase in blood pressure. Other research revealed that roughly a third of soldiers who had seen active combat had developed high blood pressure which persisted for a few months during readjustment to civilian life. Even in the dreams of hypertensive persons we see this meaningful relationship. Researchers have found more hostility in the dreams of hypertensives than normotensives.

The symptom of elevated blood pressure makes sense as part of the organism's means of furthering survival by preparation for emergency action, and other psychosomatic illnesses show similar meaningful or logical relationships. Low back pain, for instance, correlates with the sufferer's attitude that he "wants to run away." The muscles of the lower back are involved in the initiation of movement required if one actually does "run away." Chronic involvement of those muscles leads to fatigue following sustained tensing or contraction, and hence to muscle spasms and low back pain.

Similarly, other stress diseases disclose the same type of information pointing to self-infliction of these pathologic states. Dr. Graham described the attitude accompanying the crippling condition of rheumatoid arthritis as "a feeling of being tied down and wanting to get free." In hives it has been observed that disturbing life events regularly precede attacks. The skin shows irritation as if it has been physically beaten. The attitude corresponding to hives entails a feeling of "taking a beating" and being helpless to do anything about it.

The correlation between specific attitudes or emotions, and physical conditions is so reliable that physicians knowledgeable in this area can actually diagnose diseases on the basis of psychological information alone. Patients with stress diseases have been interviewed and asked key questions designed to identify specific attitudes and emotions. Although asked nothing about their symptoms, and although their bodies were visually concealed from investigators, correct diagnoses were made quite routinely.

These extraordinary findings would appear to have opened the door of scientific medicine to holism. Their implications for the vast significance of psychological factors in disease are revolutionary. They point unmistakably to a self-regulation capacity gone awry, showing illness to be something other than physical reactions to physical influences.

But Dr. Alexander and the psychoanalysts, as well as Dr. Graham and his associates, were concerned with psychogenesis. Their findings therefore carried the stigma of mentalism – a deviation from the proven course of hard science. Their brilliant analyses were consequently not sufficient to revolutionize medical opinion or conduct, and mind remains as causally ineffective as ever. Thus although individuals can be seen to produce symptoms through mental habits and daily behaviors, medicine has not rejoiced in the discovery of the "causes" of these diseases. No Nobel Prizes have been awarded these investigators and, most regrettably, no revision of medical therapeutics has followed their revelations. Medicine continues to seek physical causes for each of the stress diseases, and innovations in treatment methods continue to be physico-chemically based.

The mind-body problem has enveloped all psychosomatic disorders in a veil of mystery. To dispel that mystery science seeks physical explanations which clear the air. Physical explanations *are* lauded as scientific discoveries, and they supplant psychological explanations as soon as they become available.

In hypertension, for instance, a very small percentage of cases have known, physical causes. Most frequently, hypertension is not secondary to any known underlying physical process, but is primary or "essential." The medical world remains confident, however, that when more is known about physiopathology, all instances of hypertension will be analyzable according to underlying physico-chemical causes. Thus the psychosomatic diagnosis will come to represent fewer and fewer cases as knowledge of physical mechanisms accumulates, and confidence in the existence of physical causes knows no bounds.

Scientific medicine cannot welcome the psychosomatic disorder, as such, into its fold. This situation is likely to remain much as it is today unless revolutionary events occur. These disorders are not curable. They are poorly understood because of the mystery of psychological causation of physical events. They are, in a sense, self-inflicted but we remain ignorant of the means for remediation. They are linked to "stress" but we know not how to reverse the stress process nor even how to achieve consensus on a definition of stress itself. Finally, these disorders occur in near epidemic proportions to the extent that it is unlikely any one of us will escape their influence.

This brings us to the troublesome question of the status of the sufferer, and we inquire now into the everyday ramifications of the problem of dualism in medical practice.

b. The Sufferer and the Specialists

Since no certainty exists as to the causes of disorders of the whole, remedies recommended are as diverse as the specialities within our health care system. To illustrate how our failure to understand the whole of human nature influences everyday medical practice consider a hypothetical case of a victim of headaches.

Tom is a young man with no history of serious health problems whose occasional headaches have begun to increase in both frequency and intensity. Over-the-counter medications which formerly sufficed to eliminate the pain are now largely ineffective, so Tom consults his family doctor, a general practitioner.

Headaches, like the skin conditions related to stress, are not distinct, discrete processes. A diagnosis of muscle contraction headache, migraine, tension headache and so on, is only an approximation. Rather than being limited to a particular type of headache, symptoms overlap. The most important objective of the diagnostic inquiry is to rule out the possibility of organic disease, such as brain abscess, tumor, or other 'come-at-able' physical causes. Finding no evidence of organic disease, Tom's physician prescribes a medication for pain.

Tom finds the new medication effective but only temporarily. In a few weeks he returns to his physician with the same complaint of head pain. Other medications are prescribed to no avail and Tom is referred to a specialist – a neurologist whose diagnostic tests might identify more subtle organic derangements. But no physical cause is found by neurologic examination and Tom is referred to another specialist, an eye doctor. When Tom's visual system shows nothing out of the ordinary this doctor suspects a more obscure and rare cause may be operating. He refers Tom to a specialist in dental disorders to determine whether the problem derives from unrecognized pathology of teeth or jaws.

Finding negative results in tests designed to identify dental disorders, Tom is referred to an allergist. Here an attempt is made to see if the physical cause of head pain is something in Tom's diet or environment. Though these tests are extensive, Tom shows no sensitivity to substances tested, and months stretch into years with still gradually increasing pain.

At some point in the course of such investigations a patient is likely to be told to go home and "stop worrying" because "there is nothing physically wrong with you." But Tom is not likely to rejoice at this happy news. The odds are he may interpret the information as an accusation of malingering or possibly one of overstating his case. It is also likely that Tom may be told: "your problem is due to stress." Though this statement does not carry precisely the same implications as "It's all in your mind," it fails to bring Tom any nearer to relief from pain.

With the passage of time Tom is increasingly likely to seek assistance from non-medical practitioners or perhaps from anti-therapeutic solutions like alcohol. Friends may recommend acupuncture, chiropractic manipulations, herbal diets, therapeutic massage or hypnosis. It may well be as a last resort that Tom seeks assistance from a psychotherapist.

Over the years Tom's headaches will have been linked by medical specialists to numerous possible physical causes. His condition has perhaps by now been attributed to hormonal imbalances; to excessive head and neck muscle tension; to low blood sugar; to misalignment of the vertebrae, and to chemical toxicity. But Tom may find that explanation in terms of psychological causation can be equally diverse and contradictory. The problem may be said to derive from anxiety, from depression, from an inward turning of anger, or it may be understood as an unconsciously triggered means of inflicting self-punishment.

All possible explanations divide into two conceptual categories: mental and physical, and remedies divide along the same lines. For the most part, medically sanctioned remedies are physico-chemically based and geared toward altering functions of bodily mechanisms. Psychological interpretations may identify causes as mental or behavioral factors. A vast array of psychotherapeutic and behavior-therapy remedies are available. Never, however, will the two types of explanation − mental and physical, point to a single cause. Never will causation be understood from a unified perspective inclusive of both. Human nature has been divided into parts, and specialists in health care concentrate on those parts rather than wholes.

Headaches, however, occupying the presumably "holistic" stress-related, psychosomatic category, can be neither "mental" nor "physical" according to traditional definitions of those mutually exclusive terms. Our lack of success in treating headaches is due to the same problem responsible for our lack of success in treating psychosomatic disorders in general. We simply *do not know* what they are. This troublesome reality will be explained in greater depth in the remaining chapters of this book. For present purposes the reader need only become aware of the fundamental problem of explanation.

Consider nausea. The physical explanation which claims authority is as follows: nausea is caused by an increase in tension on the walls of the stomach, esophagus or duodenum. Nausea is thus a mechanical phenomenon, and we cannot find a place for mind in this explanatory framework. Given our modern definitions of mind and body, explanation will forever be concerned with parts, rather than wholes. Thus remediation will likewise be piecemeal and fragmentary. Medical remedies will continue to be physico-chemically based, and we will never see the significance of the potential of "the whole" for self-regulation.

Though the fact is clear that by whatever definition, mind and body are simultaneously involved in generating the stress diseases, it is body to which medicine addresses attention. Body receives the treatment, and for millions it comes in the form of drugs like valium which hold no promise as cures, and make no pretense to being such.

2. 'Real' Diseases Have 'Physical' Causes: The Failure of Psychogenesis

In disorders called psychosomatic, the bodily or somatic aspect is typically quite evident. Symptoms such as erratic heart beat and high blood pressure, lesions of the skin, vomiting, and so on, are evidently physical, and physical medicine has long claimed these diseases as its own. Other disorders, however, thought to be caused in the same way but having less visible pathology, have been classified as "mental disorders" per se. These conditions, known as "hysterical," continue to be officially listed as instances of psychogenesis.

Physical and psychiatric medicine have engaged in a tug-of-war over the psychosomatic conditions. While physical medicine has claimed them as "physical" conditions and searched for physical causes, psychiatry has also voiced a claim, for decades listing psychosomatic along with hysterical conditions as "mental disorders." Today it appears that physical medicine has emerged victorious since the "psychosomatic" classification has been deleted from the most recent edition of the definitive diagnostic manual of mental disorders.

a. 'It's All In Your Head'

"Psychogenesis," for decades believed the causal basis of psychosomatic disorders, is still accepted as the basis of conditions known as "hysterical." Unfortunately for the sufferer, hysterical disorders are the classical embodiment of the failure of explanation captured in the phrase "It's all in your head."

In the modern interpretation of the hysterical "conversion reaction," an emotional conflict not allowed free expression remains concealed in the unconscious. By some enigmatic mechanism, the mental conflict becomes converted into physical symptoms involving muscles used in voluntary movement causing paralysis, or in other cases causing malfunctions of the organs of sense. These conversion reactions are seen often in soldiers following the trauma of combat. "Hysterical blindness" may follow the sights of the horrors of war. Deafness, paralysis and loss of the sense of touch, may all be instances of conversion hysteria.

Since the instatement of dualism the prejudice of physical medicine has been that to be 'real' a disease must have a physical cause. If psychogenesis is its basis, whether it be psychosomatic or hysterical, the technologic marvels of medicine will fail to remediate the condition. Despite their more evident somatic basis, the psychophysiologic disorders as instances of psychogenesis are no more easily remedied by medical methods. Symptoms of psychogenic origin may baffle and frustrate practitioners whose trusted tools and methods fail to bring about desired results. The origins of these difficulties form a fascinating venture into medical history. The central problem was clearly evident in the age when interpretations of pathologic states were more explicitly dualistic, not yet blurred by ambiguous designations involving stress, tension and so forth.

b. Nervous and Psychosomatic Disease and Malingering

What we know today as psychosomatic and hysterical disorders have always been part of the human condition. They were not 'discovered' in recent decades, but merely reconceived and given new interpretations. The interpretation given to these disorders arising in combat situations over a century ago is highly revealing of the problem of explanation, and brings into sharp relief the philosophic dilemma which burdens medicine today.

In the many hostilities of the early eighteen hundreds military doctors became increasingly aware of a mysterious type of battle casualty. In medical literature it was argued that these strange phenomena could not be disregarded and required immediate scientific explanation. The events in question concerned damage to parts of the body, or even death, "without any visible injury or breach of parts, or any appearance of the body from whence the injury proceeded."

There were many confirmed cases of sudden, as well as gradual death following combat experience where no wounds were inflicted. One case was witnessed at firsthand by a physician. The soldier should have been with his comrades in a trench but he was not, and a cannon ball passed close by above his head. A military surgeon examined him immediately and found no visible sign of injury. The doctor observed something unusual in what he called "the state of the pulse," however, and thought it wise to send the man to the hospital. There a thorough examination was conducted and no evidence of injury was identified. Nevertheless, the patient died within 48 hours of having been "nearly killed" by the cannon ball.

In another instance a soldier with a minor injury to the arm died in the hospital after a few days from similarly obscure causes. Other injuries were reported including many cases of blindness with no evident damage to head or eyes. In one case the cannon ball passed close by in front of a soldier's face, causing the immediate loss of the sight of one eye and gradually that of the other. Another injury reported involved "paralysis of the bladder." The cannon ball passed immediately in front of the soldier's legs resulting in his inability to void urine without a catheter for nearly three months.

Another typical observation was that of loss of consciousness on the battlefield in the absence of wounds or injury. How could this and other physical effects be produced in the absence of physical causes? The answer was provided by the "wind of the cannon ball." Soldiers found lying unconscious on the battlefield were said to have been "cast to the ground" by the wind of the ball. All instances of injuries without wounds; all deaths without physical causes, were attributed to effects of the "wind of the cannon ball."

The magnitude of the problem of explanation in medicine is dramatically evident in attempts to explain "wind" injuries. Physical causes seemed absolutely necessary to account for physical effects, and even though each of them bordered on absurdity, mechanistic accounts of wind injuries proliferated.

The most broadly accepted hypothesis proposed that the cannon ball travels first in a straight line followed by a curvilinear motion. If it should strike any part of the body when its velocity has greatly diminished, instead of passing through the body it "turns round the part" in the same manner as a wheel passes over a limb.

Critics of this explanation saw a minute probability that a cannon ball could move so slowly as to roll around the body, leave no mark, and yet cause death. An alternative physical explanation involved "atmospheric electricity." Some argued that the projectile in motion picked up electric charge and shocked its victims into insensibility or death.

Another futile search for physical causation resulted in the hypothesis that the projectile in motion picked up "light substances... such as grass, shrubs, mud, canvas or part of the bedding." These substances when carried along with the velocity of the ball were presumed capable of inflicting considerable injury without leaving any "external mark."

As other scientists addressed the question, more controversy and other dubious explanations emerged. In 1812, one physician proposed what he thought "an easy and complete solution of all the phenomena mentioned as accompanying 'wind of the ball'." He presumed that the passing shot created a vacuum in its wake, causing an initial increase of pressure on the body followed by a release of pressure. This pressure change could presumably compress and expand fluids in the stomach and blood in the vessels causing rupture of both. This explanation seemed effective with regard to cases of blindness since fluids within the eyes should be subject to violent expansion and contraction.

As the reader might surmise, the struggle for physical explanation was doomed to failure. In 1813 a critic found it easy to expose the flaws in each of the proposed hypotheses. Since the injuries could not be explained by any known principles in physical or chemical science, he questioned the veracity of reports of their occurrence. He suggested the possibility that belief in wind injuries originated with seamen who "surpass all others in credulity." The matter was simple: if a physical cause could not be identified, the pathology was not genuine and had to be denied. Such was the definition of medical truth according to the dualistic metaphysic. There was no grey area in which mind and body came together and functioned as one. A disease was either physical or mental, and mind could not inflict injury on the material body, even in the midst of the ravages of war.

In 1834 a physician urged medical science: "In peace prepare for war." He stated that physical explanation had failed because the laws of physics regarding the "force and direction of projectile bodies, has been applied so imperfectly." He hoped to see injuries due to wind of the cannon ball studied in medical schools as standard curriculum with more rigorous attention paid to the laws of physics.

Thus the failures of wind hypotheses did not enlighten medicine. They did not point to the fact that something other than physical explanation was required, because there simply was no alternative. Today we have explanations which at first appear to be alternatives, but our "psychosomatic" designation only places 'psyche' alongside 'soma.' It does not *unite* the two. Modern views have evolved over the past hundred and fifty years, but we must not mistake evolution for revolution. Our continued quest for physical causes is an up-to-date reflection of the same problem, and enlightened thinkers at some future time may find our physical causes as feckless as explanations relating to the "wind of the ball."

Let us retrace our steps to determine how we passed from wind injuries to psychosomatic conditions; from mechanistic interpretations of mysterious physical symptoms to "hysterical" blindness, paralysis and so on. This evolution sheds further light of historical inquiry on medicine's central problem.

Stress Diseases Historically

The association between psychosomatic disorders (headache, ulcers, hives, etc.) and conditions known as hysterical (psychogenic deafness, blindness, etc.) dates back over a century. They were then tied by the same bonds which tie them today. All seemed to involve an influence of mind, and as such they were beyond the reach of successful scientific explanation pertaining to causation.

In the seventeen-hundreds when medicine sought a physical basis for these conditions it chose nerves as the most likely bodily substrate.

Persons with such disorders were said to have "nervous constitutions," and their problems were ascribed to "nervousness" or to "neuropathic taint." But since no physical pathology of the nerves could be found, nervousness was an unexplained explainer. It did not take critics long to recognize the contradiction. In 1859 Dr. Robert Macnish wrote: "When a physician pronounces a complaint to be *nervous,* it is a sure proof that he knows nothing about it. The term nervous, as applied to disease is merely a cloak of ignorance." Not long afterward a medical periodical published the quip: "A group of symptoms unexplained you label a neurosis, and this is rather clever for you've made a diagnosis."

Despite such criticism, the word nervousness continued in use until well into the present century. The "nervous" diagnosis encompassed three types of pathology. First came "insanity," and in this instance indications of organic neuropathology were at times evident. The case for physical causation seemed hopeful for insanity, and medical researchers attacked with vigor the task of identifying physical causes in the nerves and brain. Other nervous disorders presented less hopeful prospects, however. These were the "psychosomatic" conditions and the states encompassed by the designation "hysterical."

Our modern inventory of psychosomatic illnesses matches closely with the "nervous disorders" of the nineteenth century. These included certain skin conditions, asthma, various allergic reactions, indigestion, "nervous vomiting," headache, a number of heart conditions and other common complaints. These nervous disorders could be distinguished from conditions with organic or physical causes by several indications. Their symptoms could be magnified by consumption of coffee or tea. They could be brought on or intensified by lack of sleep and "emotions of the mind," and they were said to be accompanied by a "deranged circulation" of the blood.

The underlying relationship of "emotions of the mind" to physical events such as deranged circulation or erratic heart beat was a subject no one wished to address. When a physician had completed a diagnosis and "nervousness" was the outcome, it was time to stop further inquiry. The physician was then beyond the realm of "rational medicine," and the patient beyond hope of assistance from orthodox clinical methods. Medicine then as now, seeks underlying causes. If these are not to be found in physico-chemical processes or mechanisms they simply are not to be found at all. For this reason physicians of the nineteenth century were cautioned not to diagnose "nervousness" too hastily. A thorough inquiry might disclose a physical cause which, of course, could be treated.

If the nervous patient seemed in a difficult predicament, the hysterical patient was doubly condemned. In hysteria, nothing could be seen of the physical basis of pathology: no lesions of the skin, no disruption of normal digestive processes, no vomiting or diarrhea. Though controversy existed over the designation of a few disorders as hysterical or "nervous" per se, there were many unequivocal instances of hysteria which included blindness, deafness, paralysis and loss of sensation in the skin. All of these were considered non-medical conditions since no physical basis of pathology could be found, and Freud had not yet enlightened the medical world regarding psychogenesis.

Through no reason other than historical accident, these hysterical conditions were believed to occur *only* in women. If a male reported exactly the same symptoms, the disease was identified as a physical disorder of undetermined cause. If the victim were female, the cause of symptoms was assured. It was a certain case of malingering or feigned illness, found chiefly in women with "weakly" and "nervous" constitutions.

Since the word hysteria derived from the Greek word meaning womb, the diagnosis could apply only to females. Its symptoms were interpreted as "merely the fanciful productions of idle women of inferior constitution." In these cases "the whole energies of the patient's mind are bent on deception." Hysterical women feigned symptoms of disease because they "desired to be ill." This was, of course, no territory into which medical practitioners might venture, and physicians were advised to take no therapeutic measures except those used by military surgeons in handling "malingering soldiers." The nineteenth century bottom line on hysterical conditions read: they are maladies of the imagination.

Nervous disorders having no apparent organic basis were popularly considered "imaginary ailments." This meant simply that they existed only "in the minds of patients." Because nervous disorders tended to be chronic and were seldom fatal, they could easily be construed as imaginary. This category of pathology defeated medical science, and to dismiss it as imaginary brought a sense of relief that all was well with scientific theory.

Nevertheless, a current of discontent pervaded discussion of nervous disorders, and a sense of defensiveness and bitterness on the part of medical authorities is unmistakable. Persons with "nervously constituted minds" and their mysterious symptoms posed insoluble difficulties for medical science. Women with "fancy reigning triumphant," were said to "extract painful things felt as realities out of pure imagination." Nervous patients had "developed a wonderful capacity of dwelling on their imaginary pains and of educating themselves into invalidism." One physician wrote mockingly that nervous patients are so skilled at creating imaginary symptoms that "it is surprising they are not possessed of a better stock than they usually have." Victims of nervous disorders had "loafing habits; small mental banking accounts," and little sense of responsibility. Functional, as opposed to organic diseases involved "conscious and unconscious deception," and a "preliminary ailing tendency." Gastrointestinal disorders in particular were said frequently to be the products of "mental cultivation," and their victims were "neurotics."

The source of such antagonism is apparent in the following passage where a physician betrays that disorders of this nature defeated scientific medicine. The "visceral neuroses," wrote a well known medical authority in the late eighteen-hundreds, are:

> those recurring and inveterate states of ill health, with symptoms located in the lungs as in asthma, in the heart as in angina pectoris, in the stomach as in some forms of dyspepsia... and in other abdominal and pelvic organs. It is a familiar experience that valetudinarianism of that kind too often refuses to yield to treatment directed to the physiology of the organ where the symptoms are located.

In the face of nervous disorders medicine was helpless both in theory and therapy. Only a few physicians protested the classification of symptoms as "imaginary," not on logical grounds, however, because rationality was on the side of the dichotomy. A mental event such as a fear or a wish *could not* influence a bodily process. Yet direct experience with patients suggested time and again that these impossible events were in fact occurring. In 1895 Dr. James Putnam argued that several physical diseases revealed an unmistakable influence of mind. He would have had his contemporaries substitute the term "quasi-physiological neurosis" for "nervous" disorder.

Dr. Putnam's insights arose out of observations on patients with the severe recurrent chest pains of angina pectoris. He noted that there appeared to be "something beyond organic mischief" involved in generating attacks. These "mysterious symptoms," he argued, prove emotion to be something other than "intellectual cognition." Dualism won the day, however, and no major revision in thinking occurred until Sigmund Freud's dramatic impact was felt in the early decades of the present century. Until that time the nervous disorders were not admissible as genuine cases of pathology.

"Psychogenesis" to the Rescue

Freud and the psychoanalysts opened the doors of scientific medicine to nervous disorders via a new type of explanation. They brought an innovative perspective to human nature itself, showing the intellectual world that the human mind and bodily states could be placed in a cause and effect framework. Where prior thought made "free will" the causal potentate, Freud identified "unconscious"mental causes of action. These causes also applied in certain forms of pathology. The hysterical patient was not feigning illness through a willful effort, but was made ill through unconscious influences beyond willful control.

The psychoanalytic perspective removed the stigma of malingering from nervous disorders. The scientific world became convinced, at least for a time, that psychological causes could indeed induce physical changes. As previously noted, the argument was cemented by the finding that physical symptoms could be removed by psychoanalysis or psychotherapy. If an illness could be cured by a mental remedy it most certainly must have had a mental cause.

The impact of this new perspective became quickly apparent in health care in the military. The nervous disorder had traditionally been conceived as an instance of malingering, and official policy denied all pensions for nervous disabilities. Now, however, a more compassionate leaning evolved. To cope with health problems associated with military training and active service medical science now sought psychological causes for psychological ills. The tendency toward mechanistic explanation declined, and supporters of mechanism became converts to various psychological theories. For the long neglected and despised nervous ailments a promising future loomed on the horizon. "Psychogenesis" came to rule the day, and a new therapeutics emerged. Carl Gustav Jung, a disciple of Freud in the early years, went so far as to say that superior therapeutic results would be forthcoming if somatic aspects of such illnesses were completely neglected!

James Putnam and others captivated by enigmatic nervous disorders took up the psychoanalytic banner. Physicians at Johns Hopkins began to speak from a new framework called "psychobiology." American medicine now claimed the nervous and hysterical disorders as its own, as genuine cases of pathology, and even attempted to prevent lay analysts trained by Freud himself, from practicing psychotherapy. Treatment of the sick, they argued, is exclusively a matter for the physician, and patients who in former years would have been scolded and dismissed, were now welcomed as challenges to the new perspective — "holism." By 1930, diehard mechanists among the ranks of neurologists found themselves crowded out by psychoanalytic specialists in nervous disorders.

Although Freud was dismayed by the medical ostracism of lay-analysts, he said he rejoiced in the development of "that medicine of the future" for which one American physician, Dr. S. E. Jelliffe, was preparing the way. In a personal letter Freud praised Jelliffe saying "I favor the perspective which I believe you term Holism." And in the year of his death Freud wrote to Jelliffe "I know you have been one of my sincerest and staunchest adherers through all these years." Beginning in 1902 and until his death in 1945, Jelliffe maintained the oldest journal of neuropsychiatry in this country: the *Journal of Nervous and Mental Diseases,* through which vehicle he spread the news that psychosomatic interests were scientifically legitimate.

As early as 1922 Dr. Jelliffe was convincing skeptics that medicine had to take into account how psychic factors create and maintain derangements in physico-chemical metabolic functions and in organs of the body. He gave forceful demonstrations that bodily effects are *symbolic* of psychic factors which prompt them, and that physical illnesses are frequently precipitated by unconscious conflicts. He published works with titles like "Psoriasis as an Hysterical Conversion (1916);" "Psychotherapy and Tuberculosis (1919)," and "Psychopathology and Organic Disease (1922)." He came to be included among a few contenders for the title of "father of psychosomatic medicine."

Yet even Dr. Jelliffe was not satisfied with what he had learned concerning the mind's link to somatic pathology. He speculated that the shortcoming may have derived from his insufficient knowledge of the body side. Critics objected that Dr. Jelliffe's work told only "half of the truth," and thus the mind-body problem lurked in the shadows, concealed only by the contrasting illumination which Freudian theory seemed to shed on nervous disorders.

In due time, dualism's presence would again be made openly manifest. While psychogenesis seemed to provide an antidote for the conceptual difficulties posed by nervous and hysterical disorders, it was not welcomed as an approach to physical or organic disease. A genuine holism would surely permit mental causation of other, more ostensibly physical diseases, and another personality entered here to fight for the cause. His name was Felix Deutsch, a specialist in psychoanalysis and internal medicine. Though he had already distinguished himself as a research scientist, his lectures before the Society of Internal Medicine on the subject of "mind and body" were met with outspoken hostility. He was told that harboring such ideas was tantamount to "digging his scientific grave," and he was forced to go underground for a period.

But his interest was so stimulated by the prospect of linking organic disease to psychological causes that he soon returned to the field of inquiry which in 1927 he called "psychosomatics." He spoke of a "fusion and interaction" of mental and bodily phenomena, and with other psychoanalysts, of "symbols" manifesting psychic factors in organic symptoms.

The influence of Drs. Jelliffe, Deutsch, Alexander and others made Freudian psychogenesis the initial theoretical basis of psychosomatic medicine. Psychogenesis seemed at first to hold unlimited potential for causal explanation. It made sense of the enigmatic "nervous disorders" of the nineteenth century; it gave a causal basis for mental disorders per se, for hysterical conversion disorders, and it seemed likely to be extended to encompass a large number of apparently "physical" diseases.

Thus "psychogenesis" achieved official sanction. The term "nervous," however, had such an embarrassing history, that its use in scientific literature was frowned upon. The substitute which emerged to fill its place and to represent cases of psychological causation, was "psychosomatic disease" (also referred to as "psychophysiologic"), and the "nervous" diagnosis was heard no more.

The list of disorders classified as psychosomatic grew more encompassing as research findings accumulated. Colitis, multiple sclerosis, rheumatoid arthritis, eczema, hypertyroidism, psoriasis, and Raynaud's disease among others, were added to the tally. Each successful psychoanalysis and each beneficial outcome of psychotherapy confirmed psychogenic origin of symptoms. The question of the "why" of symptom formation had been effectively answered with the concept of symbolism and the language of the body. But the question of "how," with its enigmatic basis in dualism, waited in ambush. That question would ultimately bring down the curtain on psychogenesis, and nip the conceptual revolution known as "holism" in the bud.

The genius of Freud has had few peers in the present century. His grasp of the subject of causation was sufficiently profound to allow him to see a tragic flaw in the concept of psychogenesis as pertaining to physical disease. He saw the mystery which others tried desperately to escape by denying its existence, or by treating it with total disregard. In reference to conversion hysteria Freud stated that conditions which "involve the leap from a mental process to a somatic innervation . . . can never be fully comprehensible to us."

The lack of full comprehensibility, however, was not the only reason for declining use of psychogenesis of bodily disease. Numerous psychological theories competed for prominence, and dissent within the ranks of psychoanalysts tended to blur the picture. The argument with which Freud convinced skeptics of the reality of psychogenesis was brought into question by clinical findings. The argument stated that any condition curable by psychological remedies must have had a psychological cause. But to the perplexity of everyone concerned, it was observed that psychotherapy could cure symptoms which were later found to have *physical* causes. A case of vomiting, for instance, successfully remedied by psychoanalysis, was subsequently identified as related to a brain tumor.

Psychogenesis was never abolished outright or officially condemned by medical opinion. Instead, it gradually ebbed away and passed out of vogue. Medical reference works and diagnostic manuals which employed "psychogenesis" as the causal basis of psychosomatic illness showed declining use of the term over time and its discontinuation in the 1970s. Today the word is no longer employed in the context of causation of physical conditions, except among direct followers of Freud, the psychoanalysts.

"Psychosomatic" appears today to be following the same route toward diminishing vogue. As previously noted, the diagnostic manual of the American Psychiatric Association has dropped this listing along with the synonymous classification "psychophysiologic." These terms now appear only in the manual's index where readers are referred to a new, substitute listing. Where formerly conditions like ulcers, low back pain and headaches were classified as psychosomatic and explained by psychogenic causation, today we find these conditions restored to the status of "physical" diseases. Even the word "cause" is cautiously omitted from the manual's jargon. In its place we find the less emphatic assertion that "physical conditions are *affected* by psychological factors."

And how might these "psychological factors" operate? In this same authoritative manual we find the mind-body enigma unresolved and every bit as prohibitive of progress as it was in the era of nervous disorders. The manual states that it "accepts the tradition of referring to certain factors as 'psychological,' although it is by no means easy to define what this phrase means," and the phrase remains undefined therein.

As to "stress," the American Psychiatric Association's diagnostic manual does not employ the concept as a replacement for "psychogenesis." From various indications it appears that stress factors are every bit as ambiguous as psychological factors. The physical connotations of the word stress have camouflaged the dilemma of mind-body interaction, but at the deepest level, the difficulty remains unresolved. Despite the Freudian genius, the courageous disciples who risked scientific careers to uphold psychological causation, and despite the vast body of literature which has taken form in the past half century, scientific medicine remains equally burdened by its central problem of causation.

Summary

Let us retrace our steps through the present chapter. We began with a selection of common health problems for which medicine lacks cures. We observed three phases of interpretation of these disorders, the first of which was the nervous diagnosis of the past century. "Nervousness" proved to be an unexplained explainer, had an unfortunate impact on the sufferer, and did not further scientific progress.

Next came "psychogenesis," the Freudian hypothesis which convinced many that physical ailments could have psychological causes. Though it enjoyed widespread popularity for a time, physical causation had scientific logic on its side and finally emerged victorious.

Then, from within the realm of hard science, came "stress." Patients who would have been loathe to admit to psychogenic or nervous conditions could now display symptoms with pride. No longer did they have psychological problems, nor were they simply malingerers. Because stress was an analogy from physics, it seemed legitimate and aboveboard to suffer its consequences. An impression of physical causation was created which gave dignity to the same disorders known in recent centuries as the "imbecilities of human nature."

All three interpretations: nervous ailments, psychogenic disorders and stress diseases, disclose medicine's central problem. When we look closely we find that explanation in each case fails to bridge the chasm between mind and body. Nervousness pretends to but is soon found out. While insisting upon psychological causation, psychogenesis despairs of resolving the enigma, and stress, like the chameleon, never shows its true colors, but survives by virtue of its ability to appear now physical, now mental, and now some combination of both. The more deeply one inquires into the meaning of stress, the wider becomes the divide between physical and mental processes.

Having thus seen several of the practical manifestations of the problem, we turn now to an inquiry into its cause. The responsibility does not lie with scientists who are victims rather than perpetrators of the difficulty. To identify the source we must venture into the history of Western thought, and we must call into question an assumption which has for centuries been considered an unimpeachable truth.

III

The Cause Of Our Difficulties

> Give the automaton a soul which contemplates its movements,
> which believes itself to be the author of them, which has different
> volitions on the occasion of different movements, and you will on
> this hypothesis construct a man.
>
> *Charles Bonnet* (1720-1793)

1. Human Nature Divided

The miracles of microsurgery, the wonder drugs and technologic marvels of modern medicine, represent the triumph of scientific progress over human disease. Upon closer inspection, however, we find that the triumph applies to but one segment or category of health problems; those known to have physical causes, and when we traverse its bounds we fall into an abyss of ignorance.

In 1859, a physician writing on diseases of the stomach affirmed an undeniable relationship between anxiety and indigestion. But involvement of "mental anxiety," he noted "renders the physician as powerless a ministrant to a dyspeptic stomach, as he would be to 'a mind diseased' in the Shakespearean sense." No fundamental change in this situation has occurred in the past century, save our increased hesitancy to admit its truth.

This chapter explains how we arrived at our present position of uncertainty. Common sense and everyday observations indicate that emotional turmoil and anxiety act in the formation and progression of illness. How is it that medicine is able to intuit this reality – the so called "stress process," without evolving any means of *reversing* the process? How do we come to the unhappy position in which remedies for psychosomatic problems may in some cases further the problems themselves? It is widely known that drugs taken for insomnia may ultimately worsen the condition. Severe, chronic constipation is at times linked to over-use of laxatives. The "ulcer diet" which for years recommended milk and dairy products is now believed to increase the hyperacidity responsible for development of symptoms.

It is impossible to estimate how many futile searches have been conducted by means of medical tests and exploratory surgery for "physical causes" which were never to be found. Nor can we calculate the human suffering inflicted by the "psychosomatic" diagnosis itself; by the implication that the origin of symptoms is not entirely legitimate, and that modern medical miracles will be of no therapeutic assistance to the sufferer.

How do we find ourselves in the unhappy position where well documented observations of a number of highly significant events remain unresearched and beyond the reach of science? How can we attribute a patient's survival to a "will to live," without being able to address the nature of the influence of this factor? How is it that our conceptual grasp of psychosomatic disease is almost identical to what it was over one hundred years ago when medical science was in its infancy?

The answer to each of these questions lies hidden beneath technologic wonders; beneath multiple layers of sophisticated research programs, and concealed from view by elaborate physico-chemical theory. The answer lies at the roots, at the hard core of medical theory. It is here at the very basis of underlying assumptions that we find the source of a damaging prejudice. It is that prejudice which blinds us to the "whole" of human nature and which stifles attempts at theory building in the realm of holism.

a. Mind-Body Dualism: Origins in History, Philosophy and Theology

No philosopher has had a greater impact on the course of Western civilization than the Frenchman, Rene Descartes, who lived from 1595 to 1650. As are we all, Descartes was a product of his times. The same factors which shaped his thinking led immediate followers to accept his ideas, and those ideas have come down through the ages to be accepted in the present day as unimpeachable truths.

This philosopher's life began in dire circumstances. A few days after his birth his mother died of tuberculosis. He contracted the disease, and would have perished were it not for the care administered by the nurse who gave him his name: Rene or "reborn." In his youth he remained weakly and easily fatigued, spending long hours in thoughtful contemplation rather than at play.

In young adulthood he proclaimed himself the beneficiary of a vision from on-high. Flashes of lightning and thunderbolts inspired him with a new method for attaining truth and with a new philosophy. Yet, as we shall see, the factors shaping this new understanding were less Divinely inspired than dictated by Descartes' personality and the age in which he lived. Foremost among influences was the authority of the Catholic Church to decide the truth or falsity of ideas, and to punish those whose opinions appeared heretical.

Descartes' method involved exclusive use of rationality. He chose to disregard the evidence of the senses and to begin with no preconceptions. He sought to borrow ideas from no one, and to single-handedly define for succeeding ages the ultimate nature of humanity and the universe. He approached the subject matter as if dealing with topics no one had ever before given serious consideration. When his work was completed, Descartes had reconceived all dimensions of human nature. The Cartesian legacy is dualism of mind and body, and the associated traditions of mentalism and materialism.

History had set the stage for such innovation. The dismal age of Medievalism had given way to the Renaissance with a revival of learning and a resurrection of ancient classics. Students of human nature made use of Aristotle's contributions to philosophy and science. Students of medicine revered Hippocrates and Galen as undisputed authorities. The ideas of the ancients were held as ultimate truths, and Renaissance scholars were like dwarfs perched upon the shoulders of giants. They could see what the ancients saw plus a little more.

As the Renaissance waned, however, scholars became discontented with their status as followers rather than leaders. A schism took form dividing traditionalists from those who sought modern innovation. Descartes and his followers with insurrectionary spirit were bent upon being modern and transcending the ideas of antiquity.

Descartes was so infused with the modern spirit that he determined himself to address questions as if no one before had paid them due attention. Rather than expanding upon and refining ancient views by means of observation and experimentation, Descartes chose to employ rationality alone to obtain information. He felt certain that if properly exercised, his powers of reason could deduce truths beyond question — facts as certain as mathematical principles.

In order to proceed Descartes had to rid himself of all acquired ideas and delusions and to begin with a clean slate. He accomplished this by isolating himself in a small, dark compartment and doubting everything that came to mind. If he could doubt the truth of any idea, he rejected that idea as false. He could accept as true only that which was entirely beyond question.

The outcome of this search for truth is likely to be the same for anyone employing Descartes' method. The reader might imagine himself sitting alone in thought, engaged in a quest for truth beyond question. Would belief in the existence of the chair upon which he sat be certain? It may be an illusion, or false information stemming from impaired senses. What of the existence of the body itself? The feelings and images of bodily phenomena may be mere hallucinations, the stuff of dreams. In Descartes' age it appeared quite feasible that some super- natural being or malicious demon might deceive persons into false beliefs.

When all other ideas had been rejected, there remained but one cer- tainty, for even as he doubted, he was at the same time thinking. The reality of thought itself was found indubitable. If one questions the reality of a thought process, one is at the same time thinking, and this is all that survived Descartes' methodic questioning. He concluded: "I think; therefore I am." He could not possibly have been duped into believing this, and he was proud to accept it as the first principle of his new philosophy, the foundation upon which all further inquiries would be based. The existence of Descartes' thinking made him confident that he existed, but what more could be known of this extant "I"? There was but one definition of "I" which could be held with absolute certainty: the "I" was a "thinking thing".

Next we find the philosopher departing from pure reason and moulding his principles to conform with those of Holy Mother Church. Descartes' second step brought his innovative ideas into conformity with the Bible.

The "soul" had traditionally been construed as the basis of human life and thought, and the soul was specified by Ecclesiastic authority as destined to eternal life. As described in Chapter V, the soul, prior to Descartes, was very definitely not the "mind." Thought was but one of the faculties of this vital substance which also formed the basis for growth, reproduction, movement, digestion, and so on.

Had Descartes designated the biologic soul as the "I;" the thinking thing, he would have conformed to tradition. He would have referred to a vital substance which could perish with the material body. The problem of immortality weighed heavily on Descartes' decision to redefine the soul by equating it with "mind." He proceeded to use the words mind and soul interchangeably; to equate soul with an *immaterial* thing whose only function and only defining attribute was thought. Thus the soul became immortal because it required no association whatever with the perishable body. If anyone supposed that such a connection existed, their supposition was highly dubious since the body itself might be merely an illusion. Thought was not material, so it most certainly must be distinct from the matter of the body.

But how, it might be asked, could the body go on without a directing force? What must body be if it is wholly independent of consciousness and intelligence? What influence exists to govern its movements and functions? Descartes' answer to all of these questions can be framed in a single word: "mechanism."

As a student Descartes had been exposed to a new movement in the sciences. One of his teachers had been highly influential in popularizing the view that the body could be understood as a "machine." Former thought made the biologic soul the governor of all vital functions, but the new mechanistic view showed that these functions could be conceived in a radically different manner. Digestion could be a simple "burning of fuel," and the body's energy could be identified with the same heat which propels man-made engines.

Some advocates of mechanistic explanation claimed that chemical rather than physical factors accounted for bodily processes, but regardless of which type of principle was favored, neither perspective required the governing influence of the vital principle, the traditional soul.

The mechanical technology which had begun to exert its forceful influence must have impressed Descartes' contemporaries more than a moon landing has impressed the twentieth century. In Descartes' era such technology was startling and new. Descartes himself was particularly taken by a display of animated statues adorning the gardens at Nurenburg. These manikins moved about, played musical instruments and executed a variety of human-like actions. They were powered by water forced through pipes when passers by stepped on concealed levers.

These mechanical clockworks creatures furnished Descartes with a model of bodily movement. Though their actions had every appearance of intelligent behavior, they were controlled hydraulically. No intelligent governing principle was requisite for explaining their motions which could be thoroughly understood in terms of mechanical principles. If these same principles could be applied to animal motion, a problem of long standing would be solved. That problem was among theology's burdens and concerned the immortality of the souls of beasts.

All living creatures were traditionally believed to have souls as the basis of life and movement. If this were the case, however, and if the soul were immortal, it appeared that the beasts might have access to heaven. Some argued that such was indeed the case, and that animals had morals and actually practiced religion. Descartes' definition of human nature settled this controversy with finality to the great relief of the religious establishment. Animals were "automata;" animated mechanisms like the manikins of Nurenburg; totally devoid of intelligence and consciousness in any form. In short, animals were mindless machines.

Thus mind became the exclusive possession of humanity and the beasts were barred access to heaven. The same mechanical forces governing animal motion were proclaimed the regulators of the human body's movements and functions. For skeptics Descartes had a ready response. If mankind could construct animated creatures like the Nurenburg manikins, God could certainly construct infinitely more sophisticated mechanisms: the "beast machines."

Descartes concluded that the human body was a mechanism animated by the flow of fluids through the body's pipes or vessels. The power source was heat, identical to the heat which powered other lifeless engines. A growing body of discoveries in chemistry and mechanics lent confirmation to the Cartesian stance, and among these the discovery of circulation of the blood loomed largest. The new understanding of the heart as a pump, a simple mechanical device, was taken up and popularized by this thoroughly modern philosopher.

Cartesian mechanism made ready the way for a new kind of progress in the biologic sciences. The complexity of bodily movement could be reduced to utmost simplicity. No longer had scientists to seek a governing principle; no longer had they to come to grips with the question "What is life?" Life or vitality was no longer a necessary part of the world-picture. A conceptual reductionism would soon rule the day, and human body tissue would be conceived in exactly the same terms as ordinary, nonvital matter.

But it was not these benefits to science which led to the total triumph of Cartesianism. It was instead the authority of the Church and its sanction of the Cartesian "mind." Having no association with the matter of the body, this newly defined soul was assured immortality. The problem of animal immortality had been solved with finality. There remained but one perplexity. How could the immaterial mind influence the voluntary actions of the body?

The body was the vehicle for lust, gluttony, intemperance, sin and evil. If the human objective was to attain salvation as the Bible specified, the soul or mind had to be capable of exerting influence on the body's actions. Some of these actions, however, were evidently not related to attaining heaven. The mind need have no involvement in digestion of food or elimination of wastes. The rational will need have no relationship to the constriction of the eyes' pupils in sunlight, the secretion of saliva in the mouth or of acids in the stomach. None of these functions embodied good or evil and since they could not be the occasion for sin, they could well be designated as entirely mechanical.

Other bodily processes and movements, however, were evidently related to attaining heaven. Descartes was forced to designate these bodily functions as controlled by mind or free will, despite the fact that he had made no logical provision for a means by which this association might be effected. By the influence of mind or will the arm could be raised to the mouth to eat, or raised in anger to strike. This mind-matter connection was not permitted by Descartes definitions of immaterial soul and material body. He therefore assigned the role of go-between to God.

All of the actions which could not destine a person to heaven or to hell were said to be outside of the human control capacity. Thus respiration, digestion, the beating of the heart and circulation of the blood became "involuntary functions." On the same reasoning, the disease process and the healing process were placed entirely beyond the realm of voluntary control. They were mechanical processes utterly independent of any influence of mind.

Thus originated the "mind-body problem." Though the metaphysic seemed to set a multitude of events to order and to simplify the complex, thereby furthering knowledge, an Achilles' heel presented itself. No powers of logical reasoning, and no accumulation of empirical evidence could resolve the difficulty: that mind could not influence body was a given of the system.

As theologic motives gave form to the Cartesian metaphysic and sanctioned its establishment, theology now moved into action to resolve the perplexing difficulty of mind-body interaction. Its ally was philosophy, and together these disciplines arrived at a solution known as "Occasionalism." The principle was quite simple: on *the occasion* that mind wills an action, God intervenes as mediator between immaterial mind and the matter of the body to effect the necessary connection. Each time the will wills, Divine Authority establishes the causal linkage allowing the thinking thing to move the body. This relationship, of course, did not pertain in the case of non-human animals since they had no minds or wills and were governed in their actions by exclusively mechanical principles.

Animals were creatures of nature as were human bodies, but the Cartesian mind belonged to another realm. The mind's domain was spiritual; it was fit for heaven or hell and had no part of the "universal mechanism." Human nature with the remainder of existence was divided into two categories of entities: material and mental. Though God's power was limitless and unquestionably capable of uniting mind and body, no other type of interaction between the two was logically conceivable.

The Cartesian dichotomy led to a proliferation of dualisms. Humanity in this view was not a creature of nature but was set in opposition to it. Where ancient Greek physicians sought a condition of harmony with nature, post-Cartesian thinkers sought mastery of nature. Humanity and the rest of the animal kingdom were set worlds apart, with humans in a position of unqualified superiority. The human mind was isolated from the human body and basically estranged from the natural world. Indeed, we became strangers in our very skins, but the promise of immortality outweighed any and all such difficulties of estrangement from the natural world, and the metaphysic spread and ultimately dominated philosophy and the sciences.

b. Our Concept of Body: The Implications of Mechanism

Medicine underwent a revolution in association with the redefinition of human nature. A new hope dawned for the conquest of the physical body and its maladies. As one famous physician put it "that which is mechanical can be both understood and remedied." The body was now defined as a heat-powered engine and both William Harvey who discovered circulation, and Descartes, were lauded as monumental figures in the history of medicine.

Descartes devoted the final years of his life to science, treating among other topics, the "mechanical" functions of the body such as the eye-blink reflex. Because reason and will exerted no control over such reflexes they were consigned to the category of automatic, animal movements, for the execution of which no form of conscious awareness was necessary. Scientists who failed to concur with this reasoning were subject to the accusation of atheism. Very few dared associate themselves with the old school of thought which united consciousness with biologic functions. If mind were dependent upon organs of the body it was necessarily perishable with them too.

Mind was no longer utilitarian to the scientist, and served only to confuse the picture. Mind as immortal soul became a "spiritual and supernatural part of Christianity," and scientists dared not equate it with matter. It became unanimously accepted that "Whatever thinks is immaterial."

To justify elimination of consciousness from the subject matter of biology and physiology arguments proliferated confirming the immaterial nature of mind. Was it not true that the thought of a ton weighs no more than the thought of a pound, and that the idea of an inch occupies no less space than the idea of a thousand miles? It was concluded that no field of inquiry could unite the disparate mental and physical dimensions of human nature; as they shared no common properties, no relationship between the two could obtain.

The body was delivered to the universal mechanism, and medicine lost sight of the reality that it was dealing with a creature whose essence was in fact *human*. Previous thought was dismissed *in toto*. Aristotle was accused of giving serious consideration to "trifles," and the premodern system of medicine was disparaged as altogether "foolish." Two new explanatory perspectives supplanted the former holism in medicine: chemistry and mechanics.

In the early seventeen-hundreds, physiology was defined as "animal mechanics." It became customary to use the words "body" and "engine" interchangeably. Chemical and mechanical influences alone accounted for all bodily processes. All causes of disease were assuredly "cognizable by the senses," and the challenge for the new science of medicine was to identify those physical causes so as to be able to eradicate them.

This was, of course, no easy task for a science in its infancy. The expansion caused by increasing heat seemed inadequate as a causal explanation of all forms of animal movement. A more perplexing difficulty, however, was the distinction between voluntary and automatic movement. One distinguished physician voiced perplexity after witnessing a procession of trained elephants. These massive beasts seemed to be executing a variety of "quite stupendous movements of their own accord." If the creatures had no minds, how could this be possible? Mechanical principles did not permit voluntary movements in beasts, and science was frustrated by the appearance of animal intelligence.

The absurdity of science's beast-machines was more evident to lay persons than to those formally indoctrinated in Cartesian mechanism. The gallant French soldier, Cyrano De Bergerac, was a contemporary of Descartes. After being seriously wounded De Bergerac traded military life for the life of an author of comedies. His satire on the "soulless beast" made this aspect of Cartesianism a laughing stock for the lay audience.

In this comedy Cyrano travels to the moon and is captured by four legged creatures who naturally assume that this odd looking biped is not rational. They give him some training and force him to perform tricks for their amusement. When Cyrano encounters another human being with whom he exchanges conversation, the moon beasts surmise that their utterances are meaningless sounds triggered by forces of instinct. When Cyrano learns some of the speech of the moon creatures he is taken for a featherless parrot and caged. The protests of a faction of moon beasts to the effect that Cyrano has a rational mind are quelled by the religious establishment, and these protestors are excommunicated at the end of the tale.

The question of animal intelligence, however, was of meager concern to scientific medicine. Speculation on such issues, and even the enterprise of theory building, were frowned upon. The task at hand was accumulation of empirical facts. The mission of medicine was one of observation and enumeration of events accessible to the senses. The body was a retort or vessel to be simplified and analyzed in physico-chemical terms.

Born in 1668 in the dawn of the new age, Herman Boerhaave, was the leading figure in defining the body for medical science. His venerated hero was Harvey, the discoverer of circulation. Harvey was acclaimed as "immortal," responsible for overturning "the whole theory of the Ancients," and for founding medicine upon a "new and more certain basis." This illustrious personage had demolished the "monstrous and vain Hypotheses" which prevailed in the premodern era, by demonstrating "the Human Body to be an Engine." Boerhaave defined bodily parts accordingly as "Pipes, Leavers, Pullies, Beams, Fences, Pillars, Coverings, Wedges, Bellows, Sieves, Strainer" and so forth.

The motions of these mechanical parts were exhaustively explainable by their functions, and all functions of the body were governed by mechanical laws. Indeed, mechanical laws accounted for the production of thoughts and ideas! This proposition did not violate the mechanistic view because it operated in but one direction. Thoughts and ideas did not influence mechanical processes, but were by some inexplicable means generated by them.

Mechanism permitted no causal role for mind. A few troubled thinkers supposed that somewhere in the brain existed a mysterious third thing, somewhat like mind, and at the same time somewhat like matter, which might be able to unite the two. For the most part, however, the dilemma of interaction was ignored. It presented a challenge for theology and philosophy but not for the science of medicine.

Medical therapy was in a deplorable state of ineffectiveness and the moderns were disillusioned by contrasting successes of premodern therapeutics. Mechanical and chemical remedies, however, were the sole methods justified by the modern stance and were employed despite their doubtful efficacy. In 1705, Robert Boyle, a highly influential advocate of mechanism, described the following remarkable remedy for dysentery:

> Make the patient sit over a chair. . . perforated below, so that the anus and the neighboring parts may be exposed to the fumes of ginger, which must be thrown upon a pan of embers, placed just under the patient, who is to continue in that posture as long as he can endure it.

Thomas Sydenham, a medical authority of the same period wrote: "The arrival of a good clown exercises a more beneficial influence upon the health of the town than twenty asses laden with drugs."

The failure of physico-chemical therapeutics, however, did not destroy confidence in the mechanical model. The potential of mechanistic explanation was considered boundless, and as decades passed, medicine became even more singleminded in its objectives. In the research laboratories the "soulless beasts" furnished excellent models for the study of human disease. Medical science grew and subdivided with increasing knowledge, and where anatomy once reigned, physiology, neurology, endocrinology and numerous other specialties were founded. Mechanical and chemical interpretations ceased to oppose each other and joined forces, and physicalistic theories began to prove their worth.

Disease causation was accounted for in increasingly sophisticated physico-chemical terms. Autopsy results disclosed ever present organic derangements. The causal basis for pathology evolved from "morbific matter" to a germ theory. Another view conceived pathology as a civil war between cells. Without exception, however, orthodox medicine interpreted physiopathology in mechanistic terms. Regardless of causal basis, the disease process would proceed in exactly the same manner with or without the existence of consciousness.

The bright hope for the future seemed all the more encompassing with each new discovery and technologic advance. Hefty volumes on human disease were published with no mention whatever of mind. Events which betrayed non-physical influences on bodily functions were occasionally noted, but only to be classified as strange and remarkable medical curiosities. For medicine, the mind-body problem seemed to pose no problem at all.

The pervasive mechanism, however, did pose something of an enigma for neurology when the brain and nerves came under scientific scrutiny. The objective of brain physiology was to assign functions to that organ, and although evidence indicated that the nerves were necessary for sensation, no one had the slightest idea how this relationship might obtain.

In the premodern era various bodily parts acquired their names in association with holistic concepts. The Greek word for "diaphragm," for instance, translates into English as "mind." Other bodily organs had for ages been called "sympathetic," and the brain was said to be the "source and center" of sympathy. Under the influence of mechanism, these expressions lost their holistic denotations.

A noted anatomist of the late eighteen hundreds sanctioned use of the words "sympathetic nervous system," but stated emphatically that "sympathetic nerves have no special relation to sympathies." This same scientist gave us the nomenclature in use today which includes the term "autonomic." "Automatic" was formerly used, and pointed to the mechanical nature of nervous functioning. The new word "autonomic," extended the meaning still further in the direction of Cartesianism. Autonomous means that the nervous process goes on in independence of any external influences. It is important to note here, that this nervous system underlies all bodily events associated with emotions, and that it is this branch of the nervous system, the autonomic branch, which underlies the stress diseases.

Development of modern thought on the nerves presents a study in paradoxes. Science gave us a sympathetic nervous system with the caution that it was not the basis of any kind of sympathy. It designated an automatic, autonomous nervous system which was at the same time the basis of all events pertaining to emotion. All of this was consistent with an implication of dualism: our bodies are totally beyond our powers of control.

Throughout the post-Cartesian era, mechanism and nervous functions made strange bedfellows. As the problem of dualism was insoluble, scientists sought recourse and protection in ambiguity. The concept of irritability in particular gave scientists a false sense of security. In the late seventeen hundreds Albrecht von Haller (1708-1777) conducted extensive laboratory experiments on live animals. His influential work elevated physiology to the status of an independent science. Haller's experiments concerned the "irritability" of living tissue.

Like the word "sympathetic" with its now physical, now mental meanings, "irritability" became riddled with ambiguity. In 1826 a medical author wrote that though the word "irritation" was in "constant use," it had "no precise idea affixed to it." Irritability was adopted by persons whose views occupied *opposite poles* as to its meaning. It survived censorship, however, because of its ambiguity, and because it was made to harmonize with the Cartesian dichotomy.

Haller's definitive interpretation of irritability of living tissue was mechanistic and reductionistic. Mind was totally isolated from the phenomenon. Haller went so far as to offer scientific proof of this separation. Mind or "soul," he assumed, was located in the head. An isolated limb, however, continues to manifest irritability for a time after its amputation. If the mind were involved in this mechanical process, we would have to assume the existence of an "involuntary act of the will," or an "insensible sensation." Such an event was preposterous, so mind must be independent of the tissue irritability which causes muscle contraction and bodily movement.

Thus irritability and animal motion were exclusively dependent upon laws governing matter: "the arrangement of the ultimate particles." Haller's concept stood on the established foundation of the dualistic metaphysic. Later thinkers, in desperation for explanation, mingled mind with nerves and muscles giving irritability its ambiguous now physical, now mental connotations.

The conceptual difficulties of integrating mentalism and mechanism were most keenly felt by students of brain function. How were they to proceed without becoming impaled on the horns of the dilemma? Could they say that mind was irrelevant to brain function, or would they be forced to conclude that biochemical mechanisms *interacted* with the immaterial substance to produce the obvious facts of sensation, perception and purposeful, intelligent motivated action?

Both alternatives, however unappealing they may now appear to us in retrospect, were taken. One school of thought argued convincingly that mind bore absolutely no functional relationship to brain and nerves. This "conscious automaton theory" removed the theologic trappings from Cartesianism and paraphrased the stance for a modern audience. The "will," according to this view, had no possible influence on bodily matter. The only thing which influenced matter was the position and motion of surrounding matter. Consciousness in this view was an inconsequential accompaniment of nervous processes.

The body in the conscious automaton interpretation was to be analyzed from the perspective of physiology, and that science was defined as "mechanical engineering." As to other forms of animal life: "brutes are a superior race of marionettes." The conscious experience of humans is like the sound of the bell to the clockworks. Non-human animals were nothing apart from mechanical clockworks. They only simulated intelligence, and had no form of conscious experience. They ate without pleasure, and cried without pain.

This view was appealing because it purged science of the problem of mental influences most effectively. Biology, medicine, physiology and even psychology welcomed the opportunity to do away with the immaterial substance. In the present century, psychology as the "science of behavior" made a clean sweep of Cartesian mentalism.

Students of brain function, however, could scarcely adopt this perspective. If they could not speak of sensation, vision, hearing and so on, they would not be discussing function and would find themselves left with nerves alone. Thus they did speak of sensation, but in so doing they referred to a physiological, not a mental event. The "sensory nerves" were anatomized and detailed, and the "motor nerves" controlling movement were similarly studied. The neural mode of operation, however, was not dependent upon consciousness, but was "reflexive," automatic and mechanical.

Brain scientists spent much of their energy in the past century and a half mapping localization of function. They seated vision at the back of the brain in the occipital cortex, and hearing at the sides in the temporal lobes. They designated an interior portion as the seat of emotion and appetite, and even found locations for speech and language comprehension. But they could not solve, or even address the forbidding question of how brain matter causes mental events.

This enigma troubled early students of brain function who occasionally took a stab at the mystery of mind. One physician captivated by the enigma resolved the difficulty by questioning the nature of matter instead. Since atoms had not yet actually been observed, perhaps it was matter that science had misrepresented, and in so doing created the problem of interaction. Misgivings about matter, however, were the exceptions to the rule. Mind was the major recipient of popular abuse from several quarters, as seen in the following Chapter.

Summary

Let us summarize the influences of Cartesian mechanism pertaining to the modern science of medicine. At the most fundamental level the conscious automaton theory embodies our scientific conception of human nature. Since consciousness has no viable influence on bodily functions, human disease can be understood entirely apart from it. Science has thus been free to employ exclusively mechanistic models. Most modern medical knowledge of human disease has derived from research on animals, but engineering models and computer models are similarly devoid of mental influences.

As a consequence of mechanism there is nothing uniquely 'human' in human disease. The recommendation to treat the sufferer as other than a complex of physico-chemical mechanisms derives more from compassion than from any distinct awareness that the disease process is essentially *not* a mechanical phenomenon.

The influence of Cartesian mechanism is likewise evident in the behavior of patients who know only too well that a genuine and respectable disease must be physically based. They may thus hesitate to inform physicians that their symptoms appear only when their spouse threatens a departure. They may conceal the fact that the complaint originated in association with a financial setback or a prolonged visit from an in-law. If mental factors play a dominant role the disease is somehow less justified and honorable. It betrays human failures, flaws in character, and weaknesses we are ashamed to confess. It further seals the sufferer's fate since cures for such conditions are unlikely to be available.

The influence of mechanism has dictated the physico-chemical nature of remedies. Even when the complaint is in its very nature "mental," scientific medicine typically seeks its remedy in brain chemistry. A morose and dejected patient may be given a medication to elevate mood. A giddy and elated patient may well be given a pill to lower the spirits.

If the complaint is genuinely physical, remedies which are *not* physically based are disparaged by medical science. Our historic legacy has occasionally permitted mental influences to slip in through back doors, but when the full light of reason is shed on these they fade to near invisibility. A mental remedy simply cannot have a dramatic impact on a physical disease process.

In a word, Cartesian mechanism has given us "physical" medicine. The other half of the metaphysical design of the universe has led to the tradition of mentalism, and its impact is now examined.

c. Our Concept of Mind: The Implications of Mentalism

The Cartesian mind has posed an enigma to baffle the best of philosophers. The greatest perplexity attached to the concept was posed by its defining property: "immaterial substance." Like any other scientifically inclined thinker, Descartes preferred "substance" to "spirit." But what manner of substance might mind be if it is not material?

Observing that memories remain after experiences, Descartes likened the mind to a sheet of paper which, after being crumpled, retains lines and creases where folds were made. John Locke, another influential philosopher, likened mind to a blank sheet or wax tablet which, in the course of life experience, picks up marks and traces; the analogs of ideas and memories. Thus mind acts like a substance, but enlightened philosophers of the eighteenth century made it clear that the expression "substance of mind" has absolutely no meaning.

If it were not a substance, how could the thinking thing be analyzed or studied? The only apparent possibility was analysis of the mind's "contents." The components of thought processes could be broken down into individual units such as sensations, perceptions, memories, emotions, intentions, and so on. These then could be analyzed in terms of their mutual relationships: the "association of ideas." The thought of coffee brings to mind tea; the thought of tea provokes the association caffeine; the thought of caffeine provokes anxiety, etc. Many distinguished scholars devoted their lives to thus itemizing and analyzing the contents of the mind.

But the process of association bore no relationship to body, and the consensus among mentalists and mechanists was to keep their subject matters separate. A disastrous outcome of this intellectual isolationism was the termination of inquiry into questions of the whole, and most particularly, the termination of growth of knowledge on the subject of self-regulation. As demonstrated in Chapter V, the medicine of the pre-Cartesian era involved exploitation of many self-regulation capacities inherent in human nature. But when emotions became "contents of the mind," human nature was stripped of its capacity for self-regulation of bodily processes.

Occasionalism had at first solved the critical problem of mind-body interaction, but the solution was founded more on theology than on sound reasoning. Occasionalism gradually gave way to "parallelism" wherein the association of ideas runs along in temporal coincidence with nervous processes. In this view, mental and bodily functions parallel each other and do not interact.

Philosophers after Descartes spoke of a "preestablished harmony" which placed mind and body in "artificial union." The corporeal substance — body, and the incorporeal substance — mind, were said to require separate sets of causal principles to account for their respective motions. Philosophy accepted these substances as a "two-fold genus of beings." It specified that no productive interchange of ideas would be forthcoming between the independent sciences of mind and body.

The dominant school of philosophy held that all human knowledge was derived from the senses through the avenues of sight, hearing, touch, and so on. This assumption led to a discouraging conclusion regarding our potential to know the Cartesian mind. As we will never be able to see, hear, or otherwise perceive the thinking thing, we shall never come to know it directly.

A second disheartening implication of the Cartesian view of mind was posed by its violation of the commonsense notion that the brain is responsible for thought. A material substance composed of ordinary matter could not possibly generate the phenomena of consciousness. To resolve this perplexing issue some philosophers turned again to Divine Authority. As God was omnipotent, there existed no reason why He could not endue matter with the powers of sense, reason, and voluntary motion.

Debate on the question of materiality of "mind-substance" raged for generations after Descartes' death. Those who could not accept that the Almighty had created "sentient matter" turned to condemnation of the question itself. Since we cannot come to know mind directly, they argued, we must never hope to achieve an understanding of its material or immaterial nature.

Those addressing this question in the seventeen-hundreds remained ruled by ecclesiastic authority since their answers bore direct relevance to the soul's immortality. In the interest of self-preservation it was customary to concord with the Cartesian definitions of soul and matter thus avoiding censorship, condemnation and harsh punitive measures.

Another difficulty posed by the immaterial substance mind emerged in association with insanity. Dualism made physical illness easy to conceptualize as observable morbidity of matter. But how could a non-material being, a supernatural spirit, be sick? The brilliant author and philosopher Voltaire used this unlikelihood to point to the absurdity in the Cartesian concept of mind. "After a thousand arguments," he stated, "it will be faith alone that will convince us that a simple and immaterial substance can be sick."

The mental side of the Cartesian dichotomy led to problems equal in magnitude to those solved by materialism and its simplification of body. As illness was no longer holistically conceived, it had to be either physical or mental. Since the mental was somehow less "real" than the physical, a prejudice was attached to mental debility. Though a movement originated furthering compassionate treatment of inmates of asylums, Cartesianism contradicted a naturalistic view of insanity.

A popular variety of discussion of mind concerned its moral cultivation. Its appetites and passions were presumed embodiments of good and evil whose correct or incorrect exercise sealed the soul's eternal fate. In the Middle Ages insanity was interpreted as daemonic possession. Cartesianism gave solid reinforcement to the notion that mental ill-being was associated with sin as opposed to pathology. Indeed when psychiatry came into existence in the seventeen hundreds its initial impetus was simple compassion for the insane. It urged a removal of chains and cessation of abuses such as conducted tours of asylums for profit, and for the amusement of the general public. Psychiatry encouraged humane treatment of inmates: they were to be treated *as if* they were sick. Given the Cartesian definition of human nature, "mental illness" (as Dr. Thomas Szasz has correctly observed in recent years) is a "myth."

The most defeating implication of dualism, however, was its prohibition of self-control capacities. Cartesianism bars interaction as well as holism, and as a consequence prohibits concepts of self-regulation. This has led to a persistent trivialization of therapy based on psychological control of bodily processes, since any effectiveness of such therapy lies outside the realm of logical possibility.

2. What Dualism Forbids

a. Mind-Body Interaction and the Problem of Disease Causation

Cartesianism had a visible and dramatic impact on the sciences. The Church, however, seeing that the "universal mechanism," allowed the natural world to carry on in utter and complete independence of Divine intervention, had misgivings. Descartes had written to a friend: "on no account will I publish anything that contains a word which might displease the Church." Perhaps the philosopher did not anticipate the extent to which mechanism would be applied as the causal basis of all natural phenomena inclusive of human action.

Neither is Descartes likely to have foreseen the ultimate impact of his philosophy on medicine, since he felt that medicine might some day furnish answers as to how persons might be made "wiser and abler." Nor could he have foreseen the kinds of conceptual difficulties his system would create for future ages. Let us consider one such conundrum – the problem of interaction.

By definition no mutual influences exist between mind and body, but this flies so forcefully in the face of the evidence of the senses that many scientists have insisted upon such interaction in spite of themselves. Their violations of logic gave some "psychosomatic" concepts disreputable names. In 1972 a scientist incensed by the sullied reputation of his field of inquiry wrote that the resistance to psychosomatics was caused by:

> the non-scientific approach and excessive claims made by some enthusiastic advocates of the psychosomatic approach. This approach still seeks chimaeric connections between psyche and soma and believes that emotions 'cause' bodily changes.

Historic figures who sought these "chimaeric connections" found themselves in impossible logical straits. One such difficulty was of the 'which came first the chicken or the egg' variety. In the nineteen-hundreds it was proposed that the cause of indigestion was mental depression. It was not long before opposition arose asserting that the indigestion was the cause of the mental depression. The argument climaxed and terminated when another viewpoint expressed that *both* directions of causality pertained, which seemed to disclose the futility of the whole debate.

When a twentieth century scientist claims that a biochemical brain state causes schizophrenic symptoms, that scientist stands on no safer ground than nineteenth century predecessors. Opponents are perfectly justified in speculating that the mental problem antedates and causes the biochemical imbalance. These arguments have ever been part science and part nonsense, impossible to resolve and basically self-contradictory because they assume mind-body interactions which are themselves forbidden by the rules of science.

In a few historic instances advocates of mental causation convinced their contemporaries, but never for very long. Psychological explanation has been forsaken in all cases where satisfactory physical explanations have later been found. The longest reign of mental causes of bodily disorders was enjoyed by Freud's hypothesis of "psychogenesis."

As a student Freud had witnessed events which he construed as clear instances of mental causation of physical symptoms. He marveled at the observation that a disturbed person, paralyzed and for years confined to a wheelchair, could be hypnotized and induced to rise and walk, but after the hypnotic suggestion was removed and ordinary consciousness restored, paralysis returned.

The flow of "psychic energy," in Freud's non-physical model, explained both the origin of the paralysis and its suspension under hypnosis. The scientific community became convinced, at least for a time, that the genesis of physical symptoms could be psychological. For decades the "nervous disorders" were presumed to be instances of psychogenesis. Low back pain, headache and ulcers were listed in manuals of "mental" diseases along with the "hysterical conversion reactions" of blindness, deafness and so on, discussed in the previous chapter.

Science returned to its senses only gradually. There was no outcry or furor attached to the restoration of ulcers and other psychosomatic problems to the status of "physical" conditions. Dualistic logic has triumphed in the present decade just as it has time and again during the past three centuries. The mind has no causal effectiveness and interaction is as much a violation of logic today as it was when Descartes gave us our definitions of immaterial mind and physical body.

b. Holism: A 'Will O' the Wisp'

If all of this is true we might well inquire as to the meaning of the much touted "holism." The word has come to be associated with a variety of innovative approaches to health maintenance and disease prevention. Some are sound, scientifically based and sanctioned by health professionals. Others are dubious at best and remain afloat merely by virtue of their association with the tidal wave of popularity of "holism" itself.

"Holistic health" has captivated the lay and professional imagination and created some necessary awareness of personal responsibility. It has to a degree broadened our consciousness beyond the confines of mechanism, and pointed the way to future reform. Yet we search in vain for a fundamental definition of "holism," or for any exposition of human nature which mandates medical reform.

Pioneers of the movement have insisted that "mind and body" form a "unified whole." Small wonder that they probe no more deeply into this unchartable territory. Those who have plumbed the depths have found themselves in the unfortunate position of having to posit "mind substance, unseen energies," and a variety of notoriously undefinable "forces."

Most advocates of holism opt for the justification posed by eighteenth century reformers of medicine who preferred to treat the "sufferer" rather than the "machine." At times holism is justified in the literature by the argument that it is simply more humane or humanistic than traditional medicine, and many feel that holistic medicine should presumably work better.

A small percentage of standard medical practitioners have thrown up their hands and advised: "If it works, use it." Yet medical opinion is thoroughly justified in being conservative here. The bottom line reads "the outcomes of holistic methods are fundamentally inexplicable." Mystification pervades the rationale of causes and effects, and scientific logic is on the side of arch conservatism.

In England in the early decades of the present century a holistic movement was arrested in its tracks by the indignation of scientists. It is important to note that this antagonism was not aroused by any *ineffectiveness* of alternate healing strategies. It was widely acknowledged that these methods were quite successful with nervous or psychosomatic disorders. The indignation arose from the problem of explanation. The *British Medical Journal* summarized the state of affairs as it stood in the nineteen-thirties:

> The reluctance of the profession to adopt a pyschological outlook cannot be dissociated from the growth of unorthodox cults which continue to flourish and impress in fields where orthodox medicine often fails. Moreover, within the medical profession itself, lack of instruction in how to think about illness in an adequate way is responsible for many "good men going wrong" when, discouraged by their failure to get permanent results by standardized mechanistic

methods, they begin to adopt freakish methods of treatment which have no real scientific foundation. It is true that they may obtain "results," but to the detached observer their successes are very obviously a function of their personality on the one hand or of the magical aspects of their treatment on the other.

The lesson of history in this instance is that lacking sound scientific explanation, holistic events remain mystifying to critical thinkers. In the body of knowledge known as science there exists no place for "magical aspects." Nothing short of a revolutionary reconceptualization of the nature of the organism will give holism meaning. Until this is accomplished, and regardless of how many "good men go wrong," holism will remain a "will o' the wisp;" a deceptive and unattainable goal.

A genuine revolution in science redefines reality; closes old doors while opening new ones, and ushers in new terms for new concepts. But while "holism" conveys the impression of innovative vocabulary, it signifies only variations on old themes.

The fields of inquiry which have emerged in association with psychosomatics show, by their names, summations of parts. Where once we had psychology, neurology and immunology, we now have a special area known as "psychoneuroimmunology." "Biopsychosocial psychology" and "psychoneuroendocrinology" are among other fifty dollar words coined in recent decades. Each of these subject areas, however, makes use of traditional research methodology and operates within the confines of the established dualistic model.

The language of modern science betrays its dualistic basis and the word holism carries no meaning that violates traditional assumptions. We find dualism in the lay vocabulary when persons describe the mind and its "states." The Cartesian thinking thing has come to be conceived as a sort of empty box with flexible sides which can be narrowed or opened, closed, expanded or possibly "blown." The thinking thing's thoughts can be either "on it" or "in it," and can be retained or born in it. Those with minds like "steel traps" are better off here than those with minds like "sieves."

In all of this 'mind language' there is no holism. Modern mentalistic vocabulary fails to convey holistic import. When we are in a position requiring holistic meaning we are forced to employ the vocabulary of antiquity. With our pre-Cartesian predecessors we describe anger as a "boiling of the blood." We speak of "high spirits" when we mean more than the language of mentalism is able to convey. "Ill humored, hot tempered, warm hearted, cold blooded," and numerous other commonplace terms are direct derivatives of explicit premodern medical principles. As explained in Chapter V, expressions such as "It made my blood boil" spring from a non-dualistic understanding of human nature.

Given our dictionary definitions of mind and body and their perfect agreement with Cartesian philosophy, we are barred from formulating genuinely holistic principles. Mind and matter remain mutually exclusive. The following chapter discloses the unhappy fate of those who have argued in vain for holism during the reign of physical medicine. It further explains how scientific medicine, lest it be forced to confront its inadequacy, has perforce contrived an "invisible whole."

IV

The Invisible Whole

> Our mistake has been to imagine the total display as a mechanical clockworks, which could go on just the same for all science knows... without the existence of consciousness.
>
> *Erwin Schrödinger* (1887-1961)

1. Blind to the Obvious

An eighteenth century scholar described a man's life as "nothing more than a long series, a succession of necessary and connected motion, which operates perpetual and continual changes in his machine." The operating principle of this life, he continued, is "the matter, as well solid as fluid, of which his body is composed." When stated thus explicitly we may well be appalled by the scientific interpretation of human existence. This chapter demonstrates the development of the dualistic world-picture from which this interpretation springs. It explores the fates of those who voiced opposition to it, and the means by which the scientific world has concealed its dark secret by creating the 'invisible whole.'

a. Mechanism and the Glory of Science

In 1642, while Descartes meditated upon his metaphysic, a baby was born on a small farm in England. In adulthood he did more to reinforce the Cartesian metaphysic than has any other individual up to the present time. He was not a priest, nor was he a philosopher. He was the renowned scientist who defined for future ages the nature of the physical universe.

The reader will have heard the tale of a man struck on the head by an apple and inspired with a principle of gravitation. This heroic figure was Sir Isaac Newton. His scientific insights convinced the world that mechanical principles could describe natural phenomena so effectively that nothing in the universe would defy comprehension by these means. Mechanism would explain *all*.

The "all," however, for Sir Isaac, did not include "mind," and the omission was intentional. In order to occupy a professorship at Cambridge University one had to claim formal allegiance to the established Church. For many years Newton held such a professorship and his strong religious faith was widely acknowledged. He studied the Bible with the same enthusiasm as he analyzed the material world and its motions. In fact his theologic writings outnumbered his scientific works.

Among the questions he pondered was the distinction between earthly pleasure and this bliss of eternal reward. His mind allowed the peaceful coexistence of mysticism and the analytical breaking down of the physical world. As far as Newton was concerned, the mind was made for mysticism, the body for mechanical analysis.

Human and animal bodies moved by virtue of the same mechanical laws and causal principles, and these operated in total independence of mind. The matter of the body included an "electric and elastic" substance which "vibrates." Vibrations were carried to and from the brain along the nerves, and laws governing matter held full potential for explaining how brain controls muscle movement and all other bodily processes.

Sir Isaac Newton's "System of the World" encompassed body but allowed no place for mind. Over the years further discoveries in astronomy, physics and other sciences lent confirmation to Newtonian mechanics, and thus indirect confirmation to the Cartesian definition of reality. Newton showed his colleagues in the sciences and his friends in theology that one could easily have both: mind and mysticism in no way conflicted with a naturalistic, scientific view of the world. One could have both without self-contradiction, but never could one have anything in between. In that intermediate range lay intellectual chaos.

The particulars concerning bodily mechanisms were not spelled out by Sir Isaac. They awaited an extensive treatment by Dr. David Hartley (1705-1757), a physician who showed that the science of body was nothing other than a subdivision of physics. In a one thousand page work titled *Observations on Man*, Hartley expounded upon *the Frame of the Human Body and Mind, and their Mutual Connections and Influences.* Published in 1749 this work laid the foundation for modern approaches, a foundation strictly prohibitive of holism.

Hartley adopted the principle of association of ideas to account for mental phenomena, and paired this with Newtonian mechanics to account for bodily phenomena. Mental and material functions were said to operate in parallel and to co-relate or occur simultaneously. But Hartley did not stop here. His intuition and every-day observations suggested that mental events *caused* bodily events, and vice versa. So convinced was he of this relationship that he put forth a "Doctrine of Necessity" which affirmed an absolute cause and effect relationship between mental associations and nervous vibrations.

How, the reader might wonder, could this scientific physician assert and justify a relationship forbidden by logic and by science itself? Hartley proposed two possible solutions or routes of escape from the dilemma. One possibility was God's intervention; the other a third thing or mediator between mind and body. The latter he supposed might be "an infinitesimal elementary body, intermediate between the Soul and gross Body," and Hartley found this "no improbable supposition." How might this mediator effect causal connections? Here Hartley was quite vague in his explanation, proposing that this third thing had "some peculiar original Properties."

Hartley's other option was recourse to Divine Authority where the explanation of causation might be "the immediate agency of God." He was emphatic on the point that the soul was in fact immaterial. He "would not in any way be interpreted so as to oppose the immateriality of the soul," and he did not "in the least presume to assert, or intimate, that Matter can be endued with the Power of Sensation." Fearing opposition from the Church, Hartley insisted that his intention throughout was to "strengthen the proofs of natural and revealed religion."

Hartley's exposition of human nature settled the matter for modern biological science despite the mysterious void, the unbridgeable chasm which remained separating mind and body. The nerves were now held accountable for generating and controlling thought and action. Newton had said that a physical substance, a pervasive "aether," accounted for electrical phenomena, light and heat, and "the performance of animal sensation and motion." Hartley located that aether in the brain reservoirs containing what we know today as cerebro-spinal fluid.

The aether emanated from its reservoir and traveled along and through the nerves which "move with amazing ease and rapidity through the medium of this subtle fluid." Excitation of the organs of sense by light or external mechanical influences caused "vibrations" of the nerves which were communicated to the brain by the aether. After reaching the brain these vibrations left miniatures of themselves which constituted sensations, ideas and memories.

Anatomically speaking, the "white medullary substance" played the commanding role because all the nerves passed through this area at the base of the brain. Though later thinkers up to the present day have reassigned prominence to various anatomical parts of the brain, Hartley's basic design of mentalism paired with mechanism; human nature based on duality, has ever after reigned.

Not that critics haven't in the course of time protested Hartley's exposition, but their assaults have been warded off. They have directed accusations at the materialists' view of body arguing that live, animate matter is different from ordinary non-vital matter. These "vitalists" sought to fill the void left by Cartesianism, but they were defeated time and again by advocates of materialism.

Claud Bernard (1813-1878), a monumental figure in the history of physiology, championed the cause of materialism. With science on his side he insisted upon the "subordination of all physiologic phenomena to the general laws of matter." The existence of life in the human form in no way influenced the functions of the matter of the body. That matter was said to be "endowed with fixed and determinate, physico-chemical properties."

The triumph of physical science was at the same time the vindication of dualism. The science of physiology and in particular its subdivision neurology, were short changed in the process since mentalism and mechanism were logically irreconcilable. As a perplexed philosopher of the eighteen-hundreds put it: "the nerves appear to be necessary to sensation, though it is by no means ascertained in what way they become necessary."

Aside from occasional signs of discouragement such as these, the sciences were blind to any gross error in their ways. Their Achilles' heel was protected from exposure through a variety of formal and informal means, now discussed.

2. Factors Responsible for Persistence of the Illusion that All is Well with Medicine

a. The Terminology Taboo

For over a century after Descartes, scientists were troubled by what they called a "residue" between body and mind. The residue manifested itself in phenomena such as the bodily weakness accompanying the mental state of fear; the rapid beating of the heart in anger, and any state of physical ill-being which appeared attached to mental functions. The residue also presented itself in the presumed capacity of the "will" to move the body, where mind and mechanism must somehow effect a connection.

To explain such apparent instances of mind-body interaction several thinkers like Hartley proposed a go-between; an unknown entity with "peculiar properties." Since neither this solution nor Occasionalism enjoyed lasting popularity, science resorted to a new tactic. It chose to disregard the residue entirely, and by means of its banishment, to create an impression that no mind-body problem existed.

How, one might inquire, could science avoid the mind-body interaction dilemma while still discussing events like emotion and voluntary movement which point directly to the central difficulty? Part of the answer came in the form of semantic restrictions. It was assumed that if scientists phrased their sentences cautiously, not only would the mind-body problem be camouflaged, it would in fact cease to exist. It was, after all, philosophy's burden, and scientists ought not be compelled to carry its weight.

By popular consensus the scientific literature was purged of terminology which betrayed any weakness in the world-picture. The "soul" was the first to be excluded from scientific jargon and it was followed directly by "mind." These words had no place in biology, physiology or medicine, and early in the present century they were actually purged from *psychology* itself.

Science, the domain of materialism, fought mentalism with a vengeance. "Behaviorism," which became psychology's conceptual model in early decades of this century, showed the Cartesian mind's true colors. Former systems of psychology calling themselves studies "of the organism," had come to terms with an enemy that should have been slain.

Mind, to John Watson who founded behaviorism, was nothing other than the immaterial soul of Rene Descartes. Anyone involved in a search for truth who chose to include the supernatural in a scholarly field of inquiry committed an unpardonable sin against science. Behaviorism sought to make the study of the organism a genuine science by excluding mentalism and countenancing only materialism and mechanism. Watson correctly observed that "consciousness" was but another word for the soul of theology and that attempts to make it appear otherwise have invariably failed.

Science has long evinced a distinct distaste for the whole concept of mind, and its repudiation of mentalistic language reflects more than a desire for precision and exactness. The taboo on "will," "idea," and "consciousness" itself, has represented a need to purge science of supernaturalism. Descartes defined mind in terms antithetic to science. It meant animism, disembodied souls and mysterious forces suggesting wonder and awe as opposed to skepticism, facts and experimentation. The study of consciousness, to quote an historian of psychology, seemed to John Watson "an empty gesture in the empty air." With the banner of science aloft, behaviorism forced a choice in psychology's subject matter: mind or body.

The anti-mentalism crusade was by no means confined to psychology, however. It was apparent much earlier historically and as resolutely proclaimed in the biological sciences, including medicine. A leader in psychiatry in the late eighteen-hundreds encouraged a restriction to physicalistic language claiming that mentalistic terms were "hobgoblins" to frighten the scientist and "deceivers lurking to betray him." "Mind" was for the teachings of medicine-men rather than for men of medicine.

It became apparent that early Darwinists had committed a *faux pas* in attributing mental processes to animals. In their attempt to show evolutionary continuity between humans and lower forms they had assigned complex mental functions to animals indiscriminately. They might have fared better had they denied the significance of mind in humans at the outset!

Scientists found that even 'learning' could be studied and explained in the absence of mind. Learning was conceived as reflexive nervous processes, and multiple behaviors were thus reduced to "involuntary functions." In a major work titled *Reflexes of the Brain* Ivan Sechenov (1829-1905) wrote:

> The apparent rationality of a movement (from the point of view of preserving the body) does not exclude the mechanical nature of its orgin.

He encouraged readers to relinquish their belief that consciousness was the basis of action since all could be accounted for by bodily mechanisms alone.

Another leader in early modern physiology, Ivan Pavlov, did much to convince the scientific community that mind was irrelevant to behavior. In four hundred pages of lectures on *Conditioned Reflexes,* the basic units of learning, the Nobel Prize winning scientist devoted but one paragraph to "consciousness," while avoiding the word "mind." "Certainly," he began, "I will not touch on the problem of how the brain substance creates subjective phenomena." He wished only to impress upon his colleagues that science has no place for mind:

> During our many years of work we have never had an occasion to apply with any success psychological conceptions, or explanations based on such conceptions. I must confess that earlier, when seeking for actual causal relations...I sometimes, partly out of habit, partly out of a certain anxiety, resorted to those psychological explanations which for a long time have been considered as laws. But soon I understood that they were bad servants. For me there arose difficulties when I could see *no natural relations* between the phenomena. The succour of psychology was only in words (the animal "wished," the animal "thought"); it was only the assistance of indeterminate thinking, without a basis in fact... For the exact and systematic investigation of the functions of the higher parts of the central nervous system it is absolutely essential that the basis be laid on purely physiological conceptions (1928, p. 237).

Another eminent physiologist, Walter Cannon, devoted his career to study of the physiological mechanisms of emotion. For Cannon, emotions could not be looked upon fruitfully as "contents of the mind," and they became instead automatic, mechanical phenomena. The scientific world delighted in Cannon's phrase "the wisdom of the body," which gave figurative meaning to a concept which could not be stated literally. The appearance of intelligence in reflexive nervous processes suggested the "whole" which the scientist could not address. "The wisdom of the body" was a poetical turn of phrase which gave mind to mechanism.

In another manifestation of the terminology taboo, scientists were permitted to say that brain is the "organ of mind," but dared not say that the brain is "the cause" of mind or that mind *controls* brain. To step outside the boundaries of semantic restrictions was to make "extraordinary claims," and to risk loss of respect by the scientific community.

The taboos were adhered to in the medical literature with the same rigor as in the other life sciences. For instance, one could evade censorship by phrasing a sentence as follows: "His verbal report of anger *correlated with* an increase in blood pressure." One could not, however, state: "His anger *caused* his blood pressure to rise." It was, and remains taboo to say: "The awareness of impending danger *caused* a sudden release of adrenalin." But one may well put it in another way: "The awareness of impending danger *corresponded to* a sudden release of adrenalin."

The semantic clean-up effort ultimately purged medical literature of "anguish, torment, mental suffering, tribulation, misery, despair, agony," and such like, in preference for physic's quantifiable concepts of "stress, strain and tension." Though some non-mentalistic terms do lend greater clarity, most semantic prohibitions disclose an unmistakable "cover-up." The terminology taboo shelters the mechanistic model from criticism insofar as it perpetuates the illusion that the model works effectively. The taboo conceals an unknown which when finally seen will upset the Cartesian apple-cart, and that unknown is *the whole.*

b. Methodologic Restrictions

Science has coped with dualism as a prudent parent copes with a child's temper tantrums. If totally ignored it is hoped that the problem might disappear without further necessary action. In agreement with semantic restrictions the sciences have adopted various evasive conventions pertaining to research design, methodology and interpretation of results. The behaviorists, forsaking "thinking" as a subject of scientific inquiry, turned to "laryngeal habits" and subaudible movements of the vocal apparatus. A mental event could never be the cause of a bodily action, so "muscles" became substitutes for "mind substance" in psychology.

A new methodology was developed for researching subjects where mind-body interaction seemed ominously evident. The prohibition of interactionism created some difficulty where emotion was of interest, since the very essence of passion seemed bodily. Science could not affirm causation of bodily by mental events or vice versa, so there existed but one possible way of studying both aspects of the phenomena simultaneously. This method, known as determination of "correlations," became the scientific method of psychophysiology and psychosomatics.

In both psychology and medicine problems have been defined in such a way that the mind-body interaction enigma does not enter the research laboratory. Research design is based on the assumption that psychological variables are correlated with, rather than causes of nervous system and endocrine gland functions.

A vast body of knowledge has derived from such correlation research. Science has determined for instance that "stress," in the form of performing mental arithmetic calculations, correlates with increased movement in the muscles of the colon, and that feelings of hostility correspond to severity of coronary disease and number of heart attacks. Science knows that stressful "mental imagery" correlates with increased heart and respiration rates along with numerous biochemical changes. It has been demonstrated that distinct brain wave patterns correspond to particular mental activities, and that specific "mental attitudes" correlate with particular physical diseases.

Many thousands of studies have been performed utilizing the correlation method. Sophisticated bio-electronic recording instruments have monitored body while mind has been set to various tasks. In the design of such research, and in the interpretation of results, scientists are vigilant lest anyone confuse psychological and physiological, mental and material domains. The greatest caution is exercised in avoiding interactionist concepts wherein psychological constructs would be used as "explanations" of physiological events, or vise versa.

In the science known as psychophysiology (as in the science of medicine), there are two sets of theory: psychological and physiological. Although psychophysiology represents the closest approximation to "holism" in the sciences, it is a faithful offspring of intellectual dualism. No matter how extensive psychophysiology's research programs and no matter how conclusive their results, they cannot furnish us with a glimpse into the whole of human nature. Methodologic restrictions are the rules of the game of science. Psyche and soma are here strictly demarcated, and the whole is ruled out of play prior to the undertaking.

c. Discoveries 'Explained Away'

Unexpected findings in research laboratories can contribute to the makings of scientific revolutions. Confrontations with the unexpected cause scientists to rethink matters. Anticipated outcomes of research such as the correlations discussed above do not constitute "discoveries." As Professor Kuhn has shown in his brilliant analysis of scientific revolutions, "discovery" plays a role in the development of scientific theory only when it points to "something askew" in the old way of viewing things.

In the medical literature we find many instances of reports of the unexpected, but when these apparent "discoveries" seduce the scientific mind into the never-never land between mind and body, they are not treated as discoveries *per se*. Let us consider one such finding, the production of skin lesions through hypnotic suggestion.

If the adjectives "strange," "remarkable," and "amazing" have been applied to phenomena involving mind and body, it is a safe bet that those events have been largely disregarded by medical science. Were it not for the sobering influence of the ideas of the modern authority on hypnosis, Dr. Theodore Barber, a variety of fascinating findings would probably have escaped scientific attention altogether. Dr. Barber has endeavored to demystify hypnotism by explaining it in terms of known variables, namely a "letting go" of extraneous concerns while "feeling - remembering - thinking - imagining - experiencing" ideas or events associated with bodily changes.

In a recent paper Dr. Barber reviewed literature on hypnotically induced bodily changes and concluded that:

> The data presented... should, once and for all, topple the dualistic dichotomy between mind and body which has strongly dominated Western thought since Descartes.

Among several "amazing" findings dissonant with dualism, Dr. Barber discussed the production of dermatitis by "suggestions" that a poison ivy type plant had been brought into contact with the body. This experiment was conducted in Japan by two distinguished physicians, Drs. Ikemi and Nakagawa. They chose thirteen "sensitized" individuals, high-school boys who responded to the plant with itching, redness, skin elevations, edema, and small vesicles or blisters. Five of these boys were "hypnotized" by repeated suggestions of drowsiness and relaxation, and then told they were being touched by the poison leaf. In fact, however, they were touched by an ordinary, neutral leaf.

The eight remaining boys were not hypnotized, but were merely instructed to close their eyes. They were then touched with the harmless plant and told that they were being touched by the poison leaf.

All of the boys in both groups responded as if they had actually been exposed to the poison leaf. Twelve of the thirteen showed dermatitis reactions within an hour of contact, and the dermatitis appeared in the remaining boy after six hours. Their reactions became more severe over hours or even days, being in some cases very strong allergic reactions.

'Amazing' as these results may appear, they tell but half the story. The experimenters next reversed the procedure, used the other arm as a contact point, and instructed the boys that a harmless, neutral leaf was being used. Only two of the boys showed a dermatitis reaction to what was *in fact* the poison-ivy type leaf. When told that the leaf was harmless, four of the five hypnotized boys, and seven of the eight members of the suggestion-alone group, showed no itching, no inflammation, nor any other sign of contact dermatitis.

This type of finding, though invariably startling, is by no means new. Before the turn of the century observations of production of skin lesions by hypnotic suggestion were found easily reproducible. Rather than playing the role of scientific discoveries, however, these observations came to occupy the status of "medical curiosities." Following a brief flurry of attention, such findings have been buried in the archives and forgotten. In the final analysis, they have taught us nothing useful, nothing important and nothing new. They might indeed have taught us, as Dr. Barber presumed, that the existing dualistic model was inadequate, but no such enlightenment has thus far been forthcoming.

When presented with events that do not fit neatly into existing frameworks, a science seeking self-preservation has two possible courses of action. One is to approximate a fit: to say that "discovery X," is in reality a special case of known phenomenon "Y." Dr. Barber has argued convincingly that hypnosis can be reduced to the less mysterious appearing phenomenon of "suggestion," and this has greatly enhanced the scientific approachability of hypnosis. However, the void remains between psychological suggestion and physiological outcome. Dr. Barber is correct in his estimate that the mind-body dichotomy should topple under the weight of accumulated evidence. Were it to topple, however, we would find ourselves with no immaterial thinking

thing, and with no body ruled solely by mechanism. We would find
ourselves, in short, with nothing whatsoever. The dichotomy will be
made to fall only when a new structure is available to fill its place, and
Chapter VI addresses this future course.

As previously noted, discoveries or anomalous events can in many
instances be "explained away." That recourse failing, enigmatic events
may be explicitly denied. Both alternatives have a history of application in association with those bizarre and inexplicable performances of
Indian yogis. Where scientific explanations have been proposed, they
have concerned only the physiological mechanisms underlying these
performances. The mystery, of course, does not lie in underlying
mechanisms, but in the *voluntary control* of physiologic mechanisms.
Let us sample a few documented instances of control of biologic processes and observe their interpretations by modern scientists.

Advanced students of yoga have often claimed the ability to "stop the
heart." Medical science has on several occasions pursued these claims
with the objective of setting matters to order. Were the claims not
authentic, Western medicine might rest easier. The "autonomic,"
automatic functions might then live up to their names as independent of
mental influences.

In 1935, Dr. Therese Brosse, a French cardiologist, took portable
EKG (electrocardiographic) instruments to India and returned with a
record which seemed to confirm the claim. A yogi's heart activity had
gradually slowed to "approximately zero," and remained there for
several seconds before returning to normal magnitude. No revolution
followed upon this discovery.

Some decades later another party of scientific investigators traveled
to India and secured the cooperation of several yogis. One of these individuals showed "a marked slowing of the heart in each test," and the
wave form measuring his heart's electrical activity was markedly
altered. For a few seconds, the instruments recorded a flat wave form
indicating no heart activity whatsoever.

The investigators were baffled by this outcome since they could not
explain it even in terms of "underlying mechanisms." Other yogic performances related to cardiovascular self-regulation had been attributed
to voluntary control of *voluntary* functions. The chest and respiratory
muscles are under voluntary control, so the anomaly could be coped
with effectively by stating: "the subjects we tested do not voluntarily
control the heart muscle directly." Rather than acknowledge the reality

of a phenomenon forbidden by the established model, these investigators presumed that voluntary control of *voluntary* muscles was in fact accountable for the performance. The yogis then, did nothing that any of us could not do with ease.

By circumventing the possibility of voluntary control of involuntary functions, scientists kept their house in order. Evidence pointing to something more in human nature, something other than mind and independent mechanism, was dismissed by calling "X" a special case of "Y".

Other scientists, however, have taken the route of explicitly denying the reality of "X." At times the recorded evidence of heart stopping has been dismissed on grounds that the instruments in use were not sensitive enough to pick up traces of on-going heart activity.

In another case, evidence was obtained that one yogi could voluntarily slow his heart to twenty-four beats per minute (76 is normal), for a period of ten seconds, while altering the customary EKG wave form. This result, scientists were quick to note, was *not* an instance of heart stopping, but merely a case of "heart slowing."

It is commonplace in Eastern cultures that masters of self-regulation who have completed their productive lives, will appoint their own times of death, and in the presence of friends and followers, quietly expire. In 1957, a skeptical, Westernized Indian physician was called to a neighbor's house to investigate the condition of a yogi. This yogi who, to the physician's knowledge was not ill, had publicly announced that at 4 p.m. on the appointed day he would "leave his body."

When the physician arrived he found the yogi seated erect in the 'lotus' meditative posture. He was informed by the alarmed company in attendance that no sign of inspiration or expiration had been observed for quite some time. Skin color appeared normal, but the doctor could find no evidence of heart beat with a stethoscope, and no pulse. For four hours the yogi sat in that posture with no apparent heart or respiratory activity, and then suddenly went limp and collapsed. The doctor was uncertain whether or not to issue a death certificate, but did so after twelve hours.

One might assume that cases of voluntary *death* should convince Western science of the reality of heart stopping among other feats of voluntary control of bodily processes. Such violations of expectations have revolutionary implications for medical theory and practice. But no revolution has followed upon such reports, only the caution that

without autopsy we may never know whether such cases are in reality
instances of drug-related suicides.

The voluntary self-regulation capacities of trained meditators go far
beyond cardiovascular control, and extend to numerous other
autonomic, 'automatic' functions. Some yogis have shown that oxygen
consumption can readily be reduced by fifty percent; perspiration on
the forehead can be turned on and off at will, and negative pressure can
be created in the bladder allowing a yogi to "suck up half a glass of
water through the urethra for cleansing it."

In all such performances the Western mind sees something "un-
natural" which sets us ill at ease. Dualism is so fundamental to our
culture that our conception of nature cannot accommodate yogic feats
or any other events which will not submit to mentalistic or mechanistic
explanation. They have therefore assumed the status of medical
curiosities rather than that of scientific discoveries.

3. The Historic Discrediting of Proponents of Holism

Much more controversial than questions of yogic feats have been
issues of alternate medicine and divergent conceptions of human
nature. At various points in post-Cartesian history critical thinkers
have inveighed against the reigning model, and they have, for various
reasons, met with defeat. The scientific establishment has applied three
general catchwords to these dissenters and their enterprises: quackery;
vitalism and pseudoscience.

Quackery

The procedure of licensing medical professionals got underway in
this country roughly a century ago. In Massachusetts in 1890 a bill
went before the legislature designed to require anyone calling him or
herself "doctor" to pass a licensing examination by the State Board.
The objective of the proposed legislation was to suppress the vigorously
thriving practice of "mental healing" which claimed to employ "mind
and spirit" as exclusive therapeutic influences.

A physician at Harvard's Medical School, whose works in the area of
psychology are still revered, came forward and protested the legislation despite outspoken antagonism from his colleagues. He wrote to a
friend "I never did anything that required as much moral effort in my
life." Long after passage of the legislation this courageous individual,

William James, continued to experience hostility from fellow scientists.

Dr. James protested the medical licensing bill on grounds that the nervous disorders (known today as psychosomatic) were successfully treatable *only* by these alternate methods. He addressed the legislature as follows:

> I will confine myself to a class of diseases with which my occupation has made me somewhat conversant. I mean the diseases of the nervous system and mind... Of all the new agencies that our day has seen, there is but one that tends steadily to assume a more and more commanding importance, and that is the agency of the patient's mind itself. Whoever can produce effects there holds the key of the situation in a number of morbid conditions.

Although Dr. James could not agree with the theoretical explanations proposed by mind healers, he affirmed that:

> their *facts* are patent and startling; and anything that interferes with the multiplication of these facts, and our freest opportunity of observing and studying them, will, I believe, be a public calamity. The law now proposed will so interfere, simply because the mind-curers will not take the examinations.

As James saw it, the doctors who opposed mental healers were invoking the "holy name of science" and "blundering ahead with an air of moral superiority." The simplistic formula which then as now defines scientific medicine was exclusive use of mechanistic concepts. James felt that the doctors opposing mental healing "had no more exact science in them than a fox terrier." Yet science and mechanism won the contest with ease because logic was on the side of the mind-body dichotomy — the underlying, defining principle of human nature.

In 1894 William James wrote that the contested alternate healing strategy accomplished more with nervous disorders than has any combination of "chemical, anatomical and physiological information," and that "any set of sane persons interested in the growth of medical truth would "rejoice" at the discoveries and accomplishments of mental healers. There was no rejoicing, however, since the two perspectives were incompatible. If mind could produce changes in body tissues, the model of scientific medicine must have been wrongly conceived. The final word on mental cures was "quackery."

Pseudoscientists

The discoverers and early students of hypnotism incurred the double injury of accusations of quackery as well as "pseudoscience." If an inquirer ventures into a territory of investigation in the void between mind and body, that subject matter is not likely to be dignified by the word "science," regardless of how rigorous and methodologically sound the related research.

In its dictionary definition the prefix "pseudo" means false or sham. The discoveries of Franz Anton Mesmer (1734-1815) were officially assinged to the category of pseudoscience even during his lifetime. Mental healing was related to mesmerism and presumed to operate on similar principles. Those principles, however, being neither precisely 'physical' nor 'mental,' were not legitimate interests for scientists, and the very subject matter was by force of necessity condemned.

Dr. Mesmer, a German physician, saw disease as a state of disequilibrium which could be influenced by a force he called "animal magnetism." For a time he made use of metallic conductors to control this force, but after observing a mind-healer who made use of a simple "laying on of hands," Mesmer changed his therapeutic method. The procedures used by Mesmer evoked what came to be known as the "hypnotic state," a wellspring from which numerous "medical curiosities" have flowed.

Nervous patients sought him out and paid well to be "mesmerized." His successes were so evident that he amassed a fortune and enjoyed a large following of satisfied patients. Some who were cured stated afterward that restoration of their health was a matter of chance, so as not to incur the indignation of the learned. For Mesmer's contemporaries, antagonism was directly proportional to level of education. Lay persons accepted an interplay between mind and body more readily than occupants of the halls of learning.

Science decreed that Mesmer was the most famous and infamous quack of the century. While the committee of scientists appointed to investigate mesmerism could not deny its successes with nervous disorders, it declared the procedure a fraud. Mesmer was a skillful impostor, and nothing had occurred in his patients which could not be explained on the basis of known principles. Their ailments, it was decided, must have been "imaginary."

Nevertheless, the events demonstrated by Dr. Mesmer drew

widespread attention, and despite official condemnation, several others endeavored to investigate the phenomenon. Their interpretations were for the most part prudently confined to the dualistic model, attributing outcomes to either physical or mental causes. The latter approach assumed power of "mind over body" and thus failed to achieve official scientific status. The former approach brought the nerves into play and dignified the phenomenon with a new name: "neuro-hypnotism," from which "hypnosis" derived.

Physical explanations ranged from "paralysis of the eye muscles" to a proposed "mesmeric fluid" capable of mediating between mind and body. But hypnosis, in essence a holistic phenomenon, did not lend itself to any form of conventional explanation. Since it could not be seen for what it was, it has remained an enigmatic reflection of the invisible whole.

Vitalism

In the course of post-Cartesian history protests against materialism and mechanism were prompted in large measure by the ineffectiveness of physical medicine. In the turbulent era known as the eighteenth century Enlightenment, the sick could choose from among several dubious types of remedies. There were drugs and surgery, bloodletting and myriad forms of quackery, some officialy sanctioned, some not.

Consider drugs of the era. In 1746, the official British pharmaceutical inventory discarded perscriptions made of "unicorn horns, virgin's milk and spider webs." It retained, however, compositions of "pearls, crab's eyes, vipers and wood lice." Many thousands of deaths were attributed to excessive bloodletting, and the "machine" was evidently not improved by a wide variety of mechanistic forms of treatment.

A tradition grew up in opposition to mechanism, championed by rebellious physicians and a number of natural philosophers. These critical thinkers were convinced of the existence of another dimension of human and animal nature; something beyond mind and matter, which appeared necessary in accounting for functions of growth, movement, sentience, and so on. What they saw missing from the picture was vitality or life itself, and they struggled to include it in the conceptual scheme of things.

Some argued that even the simplest physiological processes, such as digestion and respiration, could not be explained by chemical and mechanical principles alone. Others pointed to the mind-body dilemma as justification for inclusion of vitality, since the brain, being composed of matter as defined by physics, could not possibly generate the phenomena of consciousness. Those who found vitality a necessary concept supported an intimate association of medicine and psychology. In their opinion medicine required more than chemical and physical concepts and remedies.

Those favoring this view had an arsenal of potent arguments to support it, based on rational justification as well as on the ineptness of contemporary medical practices. Their protests, however, proved futile in the long run, since what came to be known as "vitalism" was dissonant with the scientific view of reality.

The metaphysic of Descartes defined the universe and human nature *in toto*. If vitality were ascribed to 'mind or soul' it appeared pseudoscientific since these entities occupied the realm of mysticism and spiritualism. If vitality were attributed to matter, it became a superadded force, and good science prefers reductionism to complications of existing knowns. Adding vitality to matter was putting legs on a snake, and worse still, softening what aspired to being a "hard science."

Vitalism seemed ever to be the enemy of science. The stigma of "vitalist" was attached to several brilliant thinkers in the course of history. Each of them had, in various words, taught the same lesson: if we are to come to know the whole, we must transcend the mind-matter dichotomy. The addition of vital forces to material substances did not serve this purpose. Science decreed that as long as "vitalism and spiritualism" are open to question, "so long will the gateway of science be open to mysticism."

Those who strove to make visible the whole of human nature met with defeat time and again in the course of post-Cartesian history. As we shall see in the following chapter, however, an era existed in which holism reigned triumphant, and in which our so-called "vitalists, pseudoscientists and quacks" would not have appeared enemies of science. Modern theory based on dualism has contrived an invisible whole. In the premodern era by contrast, a philosophic assumption of holism determined theory and practice. We turn now to the pre-Cartesian era during which medical science and holism were irrevocably united.

V

The Lesson of History

...and it will be agreed that the customary movements of the heart are made not by mechanical instruments, or automatically, but by the living powers of sense and desire, which bring about strong pulsations in joy and curtail pulsations in fear.
Giovanni Borelli, 1608-1679.

1. The Pre-dualistic Understanding of Human Nature

When we venture into the era of premodern holism we are immediately confronted with a semantic muddle. In pre- and post-Cartesian eras the same terms have dramatically different meanings. "Soul" and "spirit," which once signified the psychobiologic essence of human nature, came to signify entities transcending nature and isolating humanity from the material world.

Strongly influenced by theology, Descartes' immaterial soul was made for heaven. God and the soul were "spirits" of another order, having no physical substrate. An amusing rendition of the modern view asks "What is soul? It is immaterial. What is mind? No matter. What is matter? Never mind." In the premodern era, by contrast, soul and spirit were the physically based animating principles of natural world.

In classical antiquity the Gods were embodied in natural phenomena. They resided in mountains and streams, sea and sky, and manifested themselves in human actions and passions. The world was alive and full of spirits. The animating principle, from "anima" meaning soul, was vitality. Soul and spirit were vital substances which performed all of the actions of animal sense and motion. "Mind" was but a short-hand expression for the faculties of thought, reason, memory, intelligence and so on, which, like all human faculties, depended upon the soul for their existence.

Since death came to the animal form with the exhalation of the last breath, the ancients chose breath or air as the fundamental vital substance. As ideas evolved from myth towards science, other elements were added, giving spirit a composition of air, earth, fire and water, and conceiving human nature in exactly the same terms as the rest of the animate world.

The ancients observed that natural phenomena were governed by a principle of equilibrium or balance where hot was tempered by cold, dryness by moisture, and so on. Well-being in the world was established by achievement of equilibrium or harmony between opposites, and it became the foremost objective of medicine to establish such balance in the human soul or spirit.

Spirit or soul was the governing principle in human nature. It was the autonomous, self-regulating controller of mental and bodily states, and it was the self or "I." Health then, the establishment and maintenance of equilibrium or balance, was in large part the responsibility of the individual. Premodern medicine sought means of facilitating such control. Foremost among these was cultivation of "temperance," a mean condition of the harmony of opposites.

2. Premodern Medical Theory

The Pathology of Emotional Arousal

In the Golden Age of Greece there was nothing fanciful in the assertion "It made my blood boil." The soul was "inflamed" in anger and the increase in heat made the coutenance "take fire" and the eyes glow red. All such physiologic signs originated from the heart where soul or spirit was chiefly seated, and from which it emanated to perform vital functions.

The heart was selected as the soul's dwelling place primarily because it 'feels' that way. As one premodern scholar put it "Here throb dread and fear, joy soothes this region; here, then, are the reason and the mind." Vital spirits stored in the heart regulated cardiovascular activity, making this organ particularly susceptible to damage through the disequilibrium involved in emotional arousal.

The state of one's health was determined by "temperament," but this was not the psychological concept we employ today. Temperament was a holistic concept and "hot tempered" meant much more than proneness to anger. It described a constitution or bodily state; a habit or behavioral pattern; a personality type, and more. It implied for physicians a course of action which, if taken, could prevent or reverse the type of pathology a "hot tempered" individual would be likely to succumb to. It was indeed more important for a physician to know what sort of person has a disease than what sort of disease he has.

Different temperaments meant different diseases, and a condition of health, regardless of one's native temperament, was a state of balance or equilibrium. The further an individual diverged from equilibrium, the more gross and evident became pathology.

The optimal state or condition of health was given similar treatments in ancient Chinese and Greek medical works. For the Chinese, the first and foremost treatment modality involved "cure of the spirit." Treatment of spirit consisted in guiding toward the correct path (*Tao,* or the "Right Way") those who had departed from "tranquility." These persons were said to have infringed upon the basic rules of the universe and to have "severed their own roots and ruined their true selves."

As the Greeks adopted temperament polarities of hot and cold (irascible and timorous) the Chinese employed the concepts of *Yang* (heat) and *Yin* (cold). Joy and anger were states of *Yang* dominance, and fear and grief were *Yin.* When hot temperament dominated, behavior became boisterous and coarse and panting respiration was observed. In *Yin* dominance persons were said to see their fates clearly, to tremble with fear and to become chilled. Both Eastern and Western traditions agreed that a person of wisdom was one in whom opposites were in harmony, and in whom spirit was preserved in a state of quiescence or equilibrium.

Ancient Chinese and Greek medicine further agreed that emotional immoderation meant "distemperatures" or imbalances in proportions of heat or cold. In states of arousal life was jeopardized, and specific alterations in the body's constitution accompanied each distinct emotion. The quality and extent of emotional disequilibrium could best be ascertained through assessment of the state of the heart. This was accomplished through observation of pulse, complexion and countenance, all of which manifested the condition of the vital spirit or biologic soul.

The ancients assumed that if an individual lived to old age he must have "exercised restraint and reduced desires" thereby cultivating a "peaceful heart" and a "purity of heart." The latter was identical to a "purity of spirit." Impure spirits were agitated, cloudy, "sooty," and they performed vital functions poorly, often impulsively, and to the general detriment of health.

The ancient adherents to holism saw illness as a violation of the laws of nature. The physician was nature's ally in reestablishing equilibrium. Let us consider a few premodern methods of prevention and therapy which capture the spirit of the holistic approach.

Therapy for the Whole

Mental and physical well-being were as inseparable as two faces of the same coin. The soul could only function in a psycho-physiologic or holistic manner and premodern medicine disparaged any method which failed to furnish a cure of the whole. The following dialogue from ancient Chinese medicine dates back nearly three thousand years and illustrates premodern transcendence of mind-body dualism. As a condition of the whole, disease was of an order of complexity beyond mere premutations of matter:

> The utmost in the art of healing can be achieved when there is unity.
> What is meant by unity?
> When the minds of the people are closed and wisdom is locked out they remain tied to disease. Their feelings and desires should be investigated and made known, their wishes and ideas should be followed; and. . .those who have attained spirit and energy are flourishing and prosperous, while those perish who lose their spirit and energy.

Unity and harmony, the whole and the "one," all of these were prized medical principles. Human nature was multifaceted, and to think of curing a part without curing the whole was utter folly. The disease would reappear, perhaps in another form and possibly in another part of the body, but would persist until the ultimate cause was eradicated. That cause was invariably traceable to the state of the soul which governed all vital functions.

Turbulence of soul could appear in disequilibrium of any faculty or in several simultaneously. Digestion, respiration, thought and all vital functions were faculties of the soul, thus correct exercise of the soul was prescribed for the salutary regulation of all vital functions. Both causes and cures were sought in the same place.

Equilibrium was the optimal state of health and it was destroyed through emotional arousal. Much of premodern therapy involved facilitating establishment of self-control. Individuals could not control external influences such as social turmoil, natural disaster, financial difficulties, deaths of loved ones, and so on, but neither were these external influences the direct, principal causes of disease. Bereavement, for instance, caused disequilibrium by captivating the soul's faculty of imagination. Imagination in turn, set physiologic functions into disorder.

Fear of death was considered a highly pathogenic emotion because its images inclined toward disease and morbidity. The emotional arousal which instated disequilibrium was a direct product of disturbed imagination. From the Stoics and Epicureans of antiquity to the late Renaissance scholars who addressed the question, we hear the same prescription. The mental faculties must be kept in order lest we fall prey to disease. Thought and imagination were faculties of the soul and, as such, could be made subject to self-regulation.

The therapeutic recommendation of the ancient Stoics was to eradicate *all* forms of emotion. The Epicureans of the same historic era were slightly more tolerant, dividing emotions into two categories, pleasure and pain, and condemning only the latter. The "pleasure" in question, however, was not associated with flighty elevations of mood or the pleasures of sense. It signified instead the absence of inquietude of soul. "A blessed and eternal being," wrote Epicurus around 300 B.C., "knows no inquietude himself and brings no disturbance to anyone else." Pleasure meant quieting the "storm of the soul" by eliminating mental content which caused the soul's agitation. In a word, pleasure was a holistic condition of "tranquility."

An ongoing state of emotional arousal was commonly understood as "self-murder." Music, wine, and dietary restrictions were often used as remedies, but over and above these stood education in self-control or cultivation of "temperance" − balanced temperament. From early childhood, education in medicine was recommended to facilitate prevention of illness or 'dis-ease.' Once disequilibrium was instated, elaborate measures had to be taken to restore balance, but if one were trained to observe the "motions of one's mind," arousal could be checked at its inception.

Emotions were products of "incorrect judgments," and could be eliminated by forming correct ones. For instance, if a craving for wealth is not tempered by reason, "the disorder penetrates the veins and attaches itself to the viscera, and the infirmity and malady manifest themselves and, once embedded, cannot be eradicated; for this infirmity, the name is avarice." An influential Stoic stated the same principle as follows: "When I see a man in a state of anxiety, I say, 'What can this man want?...This man is disordered in the will to get...he is not in the right way, he is feverish;' for nothing else changes the complexion and causes a man to tremble and his teeth to chatter, and droop the knee and sink upon his feet."

Numerous methods for training the soul were proposed in the premodern era, and authors expressed unqualified confidence that effective self-regulation was within human capability: "Chastise thy passions that they avenge not themselves upon thee. The only true standard is peace of mind... True peace of mind can be cultivated at all times, and nothing can hinder it."

Over time, treatment of the topic of pathology of emotional arousal became increasingly extensive and sophisticated. Toward the end of the reign of holism hefty volumes were published devoted to particular emotions and their symptoms. Scholarly works on the role of imagination in the disease process crowned the premodern effort. The theory was powerful enough to explain several events which contemporary theory is scarcely able to address. Stigmata, for instance, marks and tissue damage to hands and feet resembling the crucifixion wounds of Jesus, were easily accommodated by the theory of imagination-induced bodily changes.

The ancient Stoic and Epicurean recommendation to eliminate all forms of emotion was later modified to forbid only certain passions. The emotions of "content" were found salutary and included joy and "mirth," or laughter. "Contented passions" were said to dilate the heart and arteries, envigorate vital spirits, and to "strengthen all the parts of body and mind in all their actions."

As a passion of content, joy was described as "a medicine to the body; and food to the natural heat and moisture, in which two qualities life chiefly consists... For this cause Physicians always exhort sick persons to be as merry as they may, and to avoid sorrow and sadness, which being cold and dry is contrary to life, and consumeth men."

A volume appeared in 1612 titled *Approved Directions for Health*, and began with the following recommendation regarding laughter:

> *What is the principal natural means to prolong life?*
> Mirth...
> *What are the effects of Mirth?*
> Mirth enlargeth the heart, and disperseth much natural
> heat with the blood, of which it sendeth a good portion to
> the face, especially if the mirth be so great, that it stirreth a

man to laughter. Mirth I say, maketh the forehead smooth and clear, causeth the eye to glisten, and the cheeks to become ruddy.

Health restoring emotions could be instated by a variety of means. Physicians were advised to make use of these methods, some of which involved recourse to "ingenious deceptions."

3. Premodern 'Placebos' and the Power of Holistic Explanation

Both imagination and emotion could be regulated with favorable consequences by means of placebo therapy. The "placebo effect" (as discussed in Chapter VII), when re-discovered in the modern era, posed a mystery for medical science. The fact that bogus remedies could alter physical conditions was an unwelcome anomaly for contemporaries. This effect, however, was well known and routinely applied by premodern practitioners of holistic medicine.

Imagination was as much a biologic process as digestion and respiration. Thus it was recognized that:

The passions of the soul which follow the fantasy, when they are most vehement...can take away or bring some disease of the mind or body. For the passions of the soul are the chiefest cause of the temperament of its proper body. So the soul, being strongly elevated, and inflamed with a strong imagination, sends forth health or sickness.

Disease could be brought on or removed by means of the same psychobiologic processes. Imagination could instate, or it could reverse the disease process. For this reason several physicians wrote defenses of the use of chants, charms, spells, talismans and other magical remedies. "All the world knows," argued one physician, that the sole power residing in such methods is their power to captivate and direct the faculty of imagination:

which forceth a motion of the humors, spirits, and blood, which takes away the cause of the malady from the parts affected. The like we say of all our magical effects, superstitious cures, and such as are done by Mountebanks and Wizards. An Empiric many times, and a silly Surgeon, doth more strange cures than a rational Physician.

The ancients cautioned physicians to use placebos in appropriate cases only. As Plato put it, it does not befit a doctor to mumble charms over disorders which require "the knife."

The imagination-pathology connection accounted for mass hysterical disorders where contagion operated from one human source to another. The following account of the phenomenon appeared in 1577:

> Men if they but see another man tremble, giddy, or sick of some fearful disease, their apprehension and fear is so strong of this kind, that they will have the same disease. Or if by some Southsayer, Wise-man, Fortune-teller, or Physician, they be told they shall have such a disease, they will so seriously apprehend it, that they will instantly labour of it... If it be told them they shall be sick on such a day, when that day comes they will surely be sick, and will be so terribly afflicted, that sometimes they will die upon it.

An amusing account of therapeutic application of the principle involved the case of a man who:

> at the sight of a medicine, was affected as much as he pleased; when, as neither the substance of the medicine, nor the odor, nor the taste, of it came to him, but only a kind of resemblance was apprehended by him.

Such effects could not be achieved, however, unless the patient invested full confidence in both physician and remedy. If a physician hoped to impart a strong imagination so as to facilitate the "self-healing of a man's soul," both doctor and patient were required to:

> affect vehemently, imagine, hope and believe strongly for that will be a great help. And it is verified amongst physicians, that a strong belief, and an undoubted hope and love towards the physician and medicine, conduce much to health; yea, more sometimes, than the medicine itself. For the same that the efficacy and virtue of the medicine works, the same doth the strong imagination of the physician work, being able to change the qualities in the body of the sick, especially when the patient placeth much confidence in the physician, by that means disposing himself for receiving the virtue of the physician and physic.

Placebo use was but one application of the self-regulation principle – the assumption that voluntary control could be instated by a variety of means. Unburdened by duality, premodern physicians accepted as commonplace that bodily functions were governed by the self, the soul, the whole of human nature. Degree of voluntary subjectivity varied with degree of separation of a function from control by reason. Since imagination could be made subject to rational powers, it served as an effective mediator or go-between in controlling lower functions. These latter were "lower" in two senses, being both anatomically lower and more "beastly."

In the modern era a distinction was made between "voluntary" functions controlled by will, and "involuntary" functions governed exclusively by reflexive, mechanistic causation. In the premodern era by contrast, these latter were not *in*voluntary but *less* voluntary. The beating of the heart, secretion of saliva in the mouth, and other processes known today as automatic or autonomic, were believed subject to control by imagination. One could induce nausea and vomiting, for instance, by internal representation of a strong imagination of a disgusting and revolting thing. One could suppress nausea and vomiting by establishing serenity in the soul.

In the early fifteen-hundreds a physician presented an account of several instances of voluntary control including the case of a man who:

> when he pleased, could affect his body with palsy, some men who could move their ears at their pleasure, and some that could move the crown of their head to their forehead and could draw it back again when they pleased, and of another that could sweat at his pleasure, and pour forth an abundance of tears; and there are some that can bring up what they have swallowed, when they please, as out of a bag, by degrees.

These instances of voluntary control were not medical curiosities or violations of expectations of premodern thinkers. Rather, they were unusual instances of the self-regulation capacity inherent in the human makeup. That capacity explained therapeutic placebo effects as well as initial pathology formation.

4. Melancholy as a Disease of the Whole

As the twentieth century has its self-inflicted epidemic of stress diseases, the seventeenth century was plagued by "melancholy." As in the present-day interpretation of stress diseases, symptoms were known to be 'psychosomatic,' but premodern physicians required no such special term of designation. A human disease could not possibly be other than a state of the whole.

The highly injurious condition known as melancholy was neither a state of "mind" nor a state of "body," as we define those terms today. Instead it might best be described as a pathologic state of being. Melancholy was among the "Sores of the Soul" which constituted disease in the premodern era. The essence of holistic medical concepts can be captured in the words used by premodern thinkers, including the memorable utterances of the characters in Shakespeare's dramas. Let us borrow from these sources to elucidate the pathology of melancholy.

Native heat retreated toward the heart in sorrow as it did in the contractile emotion of fear, thus cold hands signified a warm heart. Although heat was stored up there for defense sake subserving a survival function, excessive heat disturbed the efficient production of spirits and caused the heart to "burn" and to "wither." When production of spirits came to a total halt, death resulted. Autopsy in instances of death from melancholy revealed "instead of a heart, nothing but a dry skin, like to the leaves of autumn."

The heart was not the only organ damaged in the disease of melancholy. Maladies proceeding from melancholy included aches in the joints, hoarseness and coughs, madness, "scabs and bleedings," indigestion and constipation, cessation of menstrual periods, and debilitation of the "principal parts" generally.

The foremost authority or "Master of Melancholy" was Robert Burton who lived from 1577 to 1640, narrowly escaping the influence of dualism. The faculty of imagination, with its causal role in generating symptoms, was Burton's chief focus of attention. Cases of blindness, deafness and paralysis, designated today as "hysterical," were instances of disorders of imagination associated with melancholy:

> Imagination is eminent in all, so most especially it rageth in melancholy persons in keeping the species of objects so long, mistaking and amplifying them by continual and strong meditation, until at length it produceth real effects and causeth this and many other maladies (1621, p. 122).

Disorders of health associated with melancholy could be averted through the exercise of correct thought and behavior. The heart was the "Domestic Oracle" which by means of arousal, signalled appropriate and inappropriate conduct. Persons of wisdom listened to and followed their hearts. Failure to act upon the heart's admonitions led to perpetuation and magnification of symptoms. Concealed love, for instance, and concealed sorrow were dangerous forms of melancholy. "Worry," it was stated, "is a bad disease," and grudges or "heart burnings" likewise wrought serious damage.

Of the emotions, sorrow received most extensive consideration since it was "the mother and daughter of melancholy, her epitome, symptom and chief cause: As Hippocrates hath it, they beget one another, and tread in a ring." Immunity from melancholy was not guaranteed even in persons with "sanguine temperaments," the type most natural and salubrious. Like other temperaments the sanguine variety changed about its mean with the seasons, and altered with maturation and with the repositioning of planets. Melancholy, like our stress conditions, was a virtual epidemic likely to affect almost everyone in the course of a lifetime.

The melancholic temperament most susceptible to the disease could not be totally transformed through correct thought and action. As one physician put it, despite a farmer's expertise in horticulture, he could never induce a bramble bush to produce a bunch of grapes.

Numerous therapeutic measures were available for treatment of melancholy. Bloodletting and purgation, drugs (including opium) and dietary recommendations along with changes of climate and environment were typical. Tranquility or contentment, however, the optimal condition of balance, stood over and above all other remedies.

How self regulation was achieved

As causation was conceived holistically so too was therapy. Physicians sought primary causes and endeavored to eradicate them. In some instances this involved direct intervention into a patient's domestic affairs. Shakespeare described the task of physicians as "To enforce the pained impotent to smile." In *The Taming of the Shrew,* Shakespeare presented a situation involving domestic turmoil. A wife informed her husband:

For your physicians have expressly charg'd,
In peril to incur your former malady,
That I should yet absent me from your bed.
For so your doctors hold it very meet:
Seeing too much sadness hath congeal'd your blood,
And Melancholy is the nurse of frenzy:
Therefore, they thought it good you hear a play,
And frame your mind to mirth and merriment,
Which bars a thousand harms, and lengthens life
(Induction, Sc. 1).

The self-regulation objective could best be achieved when life circumstances conduced to tranquility. In this regard the ancients identified as optimal circumstances a "modest fortune, and friends who are not morose, sad tempered and fault finding." They further recommended constancy or the absence of change in ongoing life events – a concept identical to an influential contemporary interpretation of "stress" as quantified in "life-change" units.

The psychosomatic consequences of domestic turmoil were eloquently described by Shakespeare in the *Comedy of Errors*. In this instance of pathogenesis of melancholy the cause involved:

The venom clamours of a jealous woman
Poison more deadly than a mad dog's tooth.
It seems, his sleeps were hinder'd by thy railing:
And thereof comes it, that his head is light.
Thou say'st, his meat was sauc'd with thy upbraidings:
Unquiet meals make ill digestions,
Thereof the raging fire of fever bred;
And what's a fever but a fit of madness?
Thou say'st, his sports were hinder'd by thy brawls:
Sweet recreation barr'd, what doth ensue
But moody and dull melancholy,
Kinsman to grim and comfortless despair,
And, at her heels, a huge infectious troop
Of pale distemperatures, and foes to life?
In food, in sport, in life preserving rest
To be disturb'd, would mad or man or beast:
The consequence is then, thy jealous fits
Have scared thy husband from the use of wits (Act 5, Sc.1).

Again, in this instance, a separation of husband and wife was one aspect of the therapeutic recommendation.

Imagination with its arousal consequences was the primary target in the self-regulation effort, and the spirit of Stoicism was repeatedly voiced in this context. Daily habits and patterns of thinking, delusions and fantasies had to be modified so as to "Secure all the Passes, and cut off the approaches and first Beginnings" of emotion. It was said that there is "nothing more Glorious nor more hard to come by than Government of the Pssions." If imagination were fully controlled, however, perfect regulation of the passions followed. In antiquity the formula was stated simply: "Wipe out imagination, check desire, extinguish appetite."

The ideal means of self-regulation involved accurate perception and evaluation of mental events, a circumspect awareness designed to nip emotion in the bud. Control was never to be totally abandoned even in cases when passion was morally or otherwise justified. In the early sixteen-hundreds an author detailed the "Art of getting into a rage:"

> The first step in losing your temper is to realize that you are losing it, for you thus have your emotions under control from the start, gauging the precise degree of rage that is necessary, and not going beyond it; you should lose and recover your temper with the aid of this higher type of reflection.

In the throes of melancholy it was necessary and appropriate to express emotion:

> For howsoever grief shutteth up the heart. . . yet by groaning, sighing, and weeping, the heart doth in some sort open itself as if it would come forth to breathe, lest being wholly shut up with sorrow it should be stifled.

Habit patterns which furthered the disease, however, had to be broken. Idleness and abnormal amounts of sleep were observed to further the disease process, as were excessive consumption of wine and social isolation. If left unchanged, these habits would further pathology in a vicious circular pattern involving corruption of spirits, the production of "ill humors," further derangement of imagination, increased melancholy, etc.

In love-sickness or "erotomania" a separate set of rules for conduct was prescribed. Love melancholy was a special case of the disease, though in its early stages it was often mistaken for ordinary melancholy. Shakespeare described an instance of erotomania in *Twelfth Night:*

> She never told her love,
> But let concealment, like a worm in the bud
> Feed on her damask cheek: she pin'd in thought:
> And, with a green and yellow melancholy,
> She sat, like patience on a monument,
> Smiling at grief (Act 2, Sc.4).

Victims of love melancholy were encouraged to socialize with other possible candidates for affection, but therapeutic recommendations of "lust and fornication" met with moral condemnation.

"Temperance" was the principal aid to reason in gaining its proper dominion over emotion. With temperance and the exercise of a "higher type of reflection," there was no limit to the amount of control one could achieve. The sequence of pathology formation operated from imagination to emotion, to constitutional imbalances and damage to specific organs. The sequence of health restoration or maintenance operated from correct exercise of human reason to control of disturbances of imagination. This brought about emotional equilibrium and balanced or homeostatic bodily functions – a holistic condition of well-being.

Neither disease nor its treatment could be conceived apart from the whole of human nature. The key to health, bequeathed to humanity in the Golden Age of Greece, consisted in "bringing under submission to thyself all that is thine own." The Sovereign Remedy, in both Eastern and Western premodern traditions, was self-regulation.

5. Conclusion

These inspiring achievements of understanding derived from the holistic metaphysical basis of premodern medicine. Holism was mandated by the fact that vital matter, the soul's substrate, was of another order of nature from inanimate substance. Holism was a given of the system. The heart was said to perform its psychobiologic functions "by the inborn virtue of its own substance." When all was reduced to its causal basis, the soul had ultimate authority. This underlying holistic principle is contradictory to our dualistic mind-matter definition of human nature, and incompatible with mechanistic explanations of body functions.

Soul had authority, not merely as the causal principle, but as the author of self-control. Though "madness," for instance, was an "affection of the brains," the self or "I" transcended brains, hearts and other organs. The whole was clearly more than the sum of its parts. In the context of endeavoring to achieve self-control, Shakespeare gave the following words to one of his characters:

> My brain I'll prove the female my soul;
> My soul, the father: and these two beget
> A generation of still-breeding thoughts.

Well before Descartes' birth, however, problems of pinning down the soul's substrate were causing disillusionment with soul and spirits as medical concepts. Medieval influences had imparted mystical and supernatural meanings to the words soul and spirit, which scientists found difficult to disentangle. Some argued that though real and material, the substance of soul was not "cognizable by the senses." The scientific mind could not rest easy with such seemingly escapist reasoning. Anatomical researches (including autopsies on live specimens) failed to find the soul, and experiments such as weighing bodies before and after death to determine the soul's weight, likewise proved futile.

As an outcome of these failures, the allure of chemical and physical reductionism became more intense, and the total victory of mechanism was assured when the Cartesian metaphysic gave logical justification to reductionism, making the spirits, soul, and vitality itself, dispensable as explanatory principles. Mind and matter would now explain all, and soul and spirit would be relegated to theology, forever banished from the sphere of science.

After Descartes, a lexicon of medical terms acquired new meanings through transformations involving loss of import. The holistic connotations of "melancholy," for instance, ebbed away until the term signified a mere state of mind. The most devastating outcome of the revolution for medicine, however, was the loss of human potential for self-regulation.

Preventive and therapeutic objectives captured in the phrase "know thyself" found no place in post-Cartesian medicine. The 'regulator' was defined out of existence, barring individual responsibility for health. Body became mechanically regulated, and the immaterial mind was helpless save to witness with alarm and dread the corruption of matter known as disease. Through loss of the self-control capacity, humanity suffered a loss of dignity, and medicine shared the adverse consequences. Where Shakespeare showed boundless respect for the profession, scathing satires flowed from the pens of later dramatists.

When premodern medical concepts were stripped of holism, nothing of lasting value remained. Imagination and emotion, as contents of the immaterial mind, became causally ineffective. The newly conceived immaterial soul, spirit and mind gave medicine nothing useful for framing explanation.

The successes of premodern medicine derived from one, and only one source. They had no dependence upon the marvels of technology. There were no microscopes, no stethoscopes, no thermometers. The era's anatomy was crude and riddled with errors, and the science of physiology was nonexistent. Yet how far they went by virtue of their possession of the whole, and how much we lost when the whole was forsaken!

Where premodern theory saw meaning and intelligence in the symptoms of disease, modern theory isolated mind from the picture and saw only mechanism. The achievements of the premodern era, when framed in terms of new definitions, lost their foundation in logic, and were interred with the biological soul, the vital spirit, and with the last vision of complete integrity of human nature.

VI

The Lesson of Modern Science

We do not take our diverging views too seriously since each
knows deep down in his heart that the other is quite wrong.
(From *Vitalism and Materialism: A Discussion,*
H. Neal and J. Porter, 1934)

Though the achievements of premodern medicine were mighty, the
contemporary holistic movement might appear to be closing ground on
mechanism and maintaining an accelerating pace toward instating a
new perspective. Can we not be content with the multiple facets of the
so-called "psychosomatic approach?" Are there not numerous titles
available abounding with valuable insights into mind-body 'relationships' in health and disease? Has not the holistic movement come of age
and established so firm a footing that future medicine will bear its in-
delible mark?

To answer these questions consider some recent disquieting reactions to the "Type A behavior" concept. This concept has enjoyed so
much favorable publicity to date that many business executives are at-
tempting to cultivate "Type B behavior" patterns. The public appears to
have become thoroughly convinced that health of the heart is a matter
of more than physical mechanism. In the laboratories of
psychosomatics, vigorous research programs are aimed at detailing the
coronary-prone Type A personality, and one of the discoverers of the
phenomenon has followed through with another popular title: *Treating
Type A Behavior and Your Heart* (Friedman and Ulmer, 1984).

Outside the area of psychosomatics, however, and beyond the reach
of the lay audience, words of caution are being voiced by more conservative traditionalists. In the *New England Journal of Medicine,* the
type A hypothesis was (as opponents of psychosomatic concepts have
been wont to say), "put to scientific test," and the results were "not conclusive." The researcher, Dr. Robert Case, claimed to have found "no
significant correlation" between deaths from heart attack and behavior
type. The doctor's conclusion strikes a familiar cord in modern medical
history: physical factors *alone* can be identified as leading to heart attacks. We may be assured that once identified, physical factors will be
given preference by scientists today as they have been for the past three
centuries.

A non-medical author writing in a recent issue of the *Wall Street Journal* lets us know that members of the general public also have certain reservations. It appears to this critic that publications on the Type A personality "eschew the scientific approach." Furthermore, he writes, these books "peddle the hoary folk superstition that strain can kill you."

It is not a simple, misguided prejudice which fuels such opposition to non-physical causal variables. However painful the confrontation may be, we must acknowledge the fact that sound logic is wholly on the side of critics of would-be holistic concepts. For this reason we must avail ourselves of a lesson of modern science, or more precisely, the lesson taught by contemporary physicists regarding the flaw in the underlying world-view which dictates that sound logic. This chapter is directed at explicating the flaw so as to make evident the necessity for a redefinition of human nature. Only through this avenue will a meaningful concept of holism be achieved.

Holism Has Not Come of Age

As the reader has observed in previous chapters, psychosomatic perspectives have had their 'ins and outs;' temporary vogues have been routinely followed by harsh awakenings. It might be accurate to say that present-day medicine is enlightened regarding the undeniable influence of para-physical factors in health and disease. Perhaps it knows its destination, but the route which might lead there remains uncharted, and pitfalls encumber free passage.

For a time, the Freudian hypothesis of psychogenesis promised to lead medicine to the aspired achievement of holism. But psychogenesis was not a legitimate offspring of traditional medicine, and as early as 1950 its fundamental incompatibility with physical medicine was recognized. Psychogenesis was replaced by an imprecise concept of multicausality wherein social, environmental, behavioral and stress factors were all welcomed into play, obscuring the difficulty of explaining basic causal mechanisms.

The fact remains that the bottom line on causation reads the same in the 1980's as it did in the 1950's when holism in the form of psychogenesis was defeated by dualism. The psychosomatic approach survives today because it does not posit a direct causal association between mind and matter. It is *not* asserted that social, psychological and stress variables cause ulcers, heart attacks and so on. Rather, it is acknowledged that other bodily mechanisms *mediate* and act as direct causes. Nervous processes and endocrine gland functions are still believed to be the sole immediate causes of ulcers, heart attacks and so on.

Since physical mechanisms are assumed both necessary and sufficient causes of such illnesses, today's psychosomatic perspective *is* a legitimate offspring of traditional medicine. The movement stands on solid ground since it evades a violation of logic. If it is fully compatible with dualism, however, to what degree does this perspective represent holism?

Modern holism is something of a humbug which promises much that is new and revolutionary but delivers little more than traditional products in innovative wrappings. Upon close inspection, the theoretical underpinning of psychosomatics is found to be dualism. The perspective has engendered needed reform but nothing which might be called revolution. Holistic therapeutic innovations have not become a part of medicine proper.

The neuroendocrine mediators between psychosocial factors and physical diseases establish the hook-up at the matter end of the causal chain, but this merely places us one step removed from the dilemma. Genuine holism will never be achieved by adding mind to matter. Scientific medicine's "brass tacks" are physical entities and processes. If we cannot look to bodily matter and find holism, true holism will never be achieved, and medical science will remain out of step with the human condition.

1. The Laws of Matter Can't Explain Mind

That the laws of matter can't explain mind is a given of the established system. Physics' laws do not pretend to furnish understanding here, nor could they. It is paradoxical then, that prevalent opinion within lay and scientific communities holds that the matter of the brain somehow generates the phenomena of consciousness, while at the same time, brain matter is presumed governed by laws pertaining to the ultimate particles, that is, by the laws of physics.

In pre-Cartesian theory (discussed in the previous chapter), matter generated mind by virtue of the fact that it was fundamentally different from matter found in the inanimate world. The vital substance or spirit was by definition equipped for performance of its functions. The biologic soul or spirit was a great integrator of organismic functions. It imparted sentience and intelligence to animate forms of matter whose internal spring was vitality.

The mechanistic conception which replaced vital spirit in the modern era derived from the discovery of a new form of energy. In 1792 Luigi Galvani and Allesandro Volta observed this energy in the muscle and attached nerve in the leg of a frog. Eventually, the energy understood to cause muscle contraction came to be called "electricity." Electric currents were said to travel from the brain down the spinal column and out to the muscles. The spirits had been presumed to operate in the same way, but with one cardinal distinction – electricity was not vital, and could be neither sentient nor intelligent.

One hundred years passed before Galvani's and Volta's discovery was subject to exploration through the experiemental methods of science. Research on brain function led to the conclusion that two pathways emanated from the central organ – one was described as the "Path of the Reflexes" or automatic functions, and the other as the "Path of the Will." This preserved the Cartesian assumption that mind governed only purposeful action, and mind was by some unknown means associated with the generalized functioning of the brain as a whole.

Increasing knowledge concerning electrical properties of the brain corresponded to decreasing holistic understanding of function. The notion that mind, soul or spirit was somehow manifest as the general functioning of the total action of the brain was eclipsed by mechanistic reductionism. By 1900 it was unanimously accepted that the brain operates by "isolated mechanical means." Scientists interested in elucidating brain function sought only mechanisms, and the explanatory principle evolved from electrical, to electro-chemical function. To the satisfaction and relief of scientists, mind was totally excluded from the causal framework.

Neuro-scientists had much to occupy their attention and seldom had misgivings concerning the potential of mechanistic explanation. Modern trend setters and leaders in the field occasionally voiced perplexity or irritation about the problem of dualism. Wilder Penfield, who gave us much of what is known today on the disease of epilepsy, complained that the "riddle of how brain and mind do interact is still unsolved." He resigned himself to using the "language of dualism," saying that "as scientists, we should reserve judgment as to the ultimate nature of things (1972, p. 309)."

A number of leading physicists, however, have not exercised such reserve, and have demonstrated that the ultimate nature of things is not what it has been presumed to be. They have made public an obvious and very serious flaw with an effect similar to that of the child's proclamation in *The Emperor's New Clothes*. They have forced us to an open confrontation with a highly embarrassing truth: no physical process can possibly account for the phenomena of consciousness, and science has for three centuries propagated a mass delusion.

The Nobel Prize winning physicist Eugene Wigner (1967) used quantum mechanics equations to prove that existing assumptions are unfounded. What we know as "consciousness" can be shown to influence the physico-chemical substrate − brain, and this is a clear violation of the laws of physics. Wigner concluded from this that the mind-body relationship has no analogue in the material world, and our world-picture is therefore subject to question. Wigner identified our view of matter as the source of the difficulty, since ordinary matter is incompatible with the facts of consciousness.

It has long been anticipated that the ultimate laws of matter would explain all, and that the brain of a human thinker would be fully analyzed in such terms. Today it is known that the laws governing matter as presently conceived will only continue to bar all that is mental from the scientific picture of the real world. The brain, it appears, is not equipped for thinking. Physicists have found it fitting to make public this paradox despite the fact that three hundred years of effort went into concealing it. The incompatibility of mind and mechanism is no more, and no less than the legacy of Cartesian dualism.

2. The Laws of Physics Can't Explain Vital Matter

It has also been ascertained that this problem of accounting for mind is a derivative of a more fundamental difficulty. The laws of physics cannot account for the behavior of the matter of living tissue. Science has assumed that increasing knowledge of the operations of atoms and molecules within the cell would someday render laws of physics fully applicable to vital matter. The Nobel Laureate Erwin Schrödinger (1933) has eloquently and with finality shown this assumption to be false.

The confidence of scientists was for many years falsely sustained by expectations which have recently been disconfirmed. Not only do events within the living cell resist explanation by the laws of matter, it is also known that were living cells governed by such laws, the hereditary code, and life itself would be promptly destroyed. In proving these points science has wielded its most formidable weapon – mathematical proofs. A falsehood has been disclosed and an era has ended.

Though fascinating, the arguments leading to these unsettling conclusions cannot be reproduced here, and the interested reader might refer to the primary sources listed as References. Of greater importance for inclusion in the present context is the message of hope deriving from the fact that a new perspective is taking form, one which may prove of vast significance for the future of medicine since it entails a redefinition of the nature of living matter, and prepares the way for a redefinition of human nature.

3. Reality Requires a Third Dimension

No known principles of physical science can account for the existence of sentience or consciousness in living organisms. Known principles of physics have proven incompatible with, and inappropriate for explaining the behavior of living matter within the cell.

These two problems have a common cause and a common solution. The cause is clearly the Cartesian dichotomy which has reduced the material universe, including the human brain, to the mechanical operations of the "ultimate particles." The solution to both problems comes with the realization that these particles are not as 'ultimate' as modern science has assumed, or to put it differently, there exists another dimension of reality not provided for in the Cartesian mind-matter scheme of things. Vital matter has unique properties and requires its own set of laws, laws which must also provide for native intelligence, sensation, perception, in a word, for mind itself.

The conflict between vitalism and mechanism has revolved around the issue of causation. The vitalists in post-Cartesian history have singled out events to which mechanistic causation could not apply. The existence of consciousness, for instance, was long recognized as problematic. The vitalists have said that given such events, matter in its living state must be possessed of a force which seizes upon it and exerts control while the organism is alive. The materialists have recoiled at the prospect of admitting mysterious forces, and have asserted with confidence that future physical science holds all of the answers. The life science of biology would some day become a sort of "superphysics," and biologic knowledge could aspire to no firmer foundation in reality than the atoms and molecules comprising all substances in the universe.

Reality, however, we have observed to be *relative* to time and place. A radically different reality was perceived by pre-modern thinkers for whom the true self was a biologic spirit. Materialism and vitalism defined different ultimate realities, the former compatible with Cartesianism, the latter incompatible with the quest of science. Harking back to the quotation heading this chapter, we find that we need not take the diverging views of vitalists *or* materialists too seriously. We are instead forced to conclude that both approaches have been quite wrong.

Since living matter violates the laws of physics we are compelled to posit another set of laws pertaining to vital substances and processes. Rather than adding-on a super-physical force repugnant to science, we are inclined to choose the alternative proposed by another physicist – Walter M. Elsasser. In *Atom and Organism* (1966) Elsasser explained how biologic theory must be built given that the laws of physics cannot explain vital matter.

Elsasser, with Wigner and others, convinces us that a third dimension of reality is absolutely necessary on logical grounds. These scientists have concluded that life is a primary phenomenon, irreducible to mind or mechanism, and they call this new realm the "biotonic phase" of existence. Physicists have been forced to this conclusion, not by the mind-body problem which, for the most part, was never brought into consideration. The conclusion has been forced by matter problems alone!

The usefulness of the biotonic phase concept for psychology and medicine cannot be overestimated. It furnishes a domain for the whole and opens an avenue for causal explanation which could not otherwise be achieved. Recent work by Dr. Walter Weimer has already demonstrated how the biotonic phase concept resolves our perennial problem of causation. It disempowers the dualism dilemma and dissipates the enigma of mind-body interaction since such interaction is no longer required. The causal substrate of organismic functions becomes the biotonic dimension of existence.

The biotonic phase is a frontier for several sciences and poses an unparalleled challenge. In medicine it spells revolution, gives potential meaning to holism, and lends logical justification to innovative treatment modalities which seem incongruous in the dualistic framework. Those perplexing instances in which mind appears to cause changes in body become instances of a different type of causation operating from the whole outward.

Yet if medicine has for three centuries scarcely been aware of any difficulty, why should we presume that an innovation in biology or physics should revolutionize traditional medicine? As seen in the previous chapters, the difficulty has been well concealed, and medicine has maintained unqualified confidence in its conceptual model. If we know where to look, however, the central difficulty will not remain camouflaged, but will loom large and menacing.

In the fables of India we find the tale of a clever jackal who made visible a concealed problem. A hungry lion had hidden in the jackal's cave and waited there to devour him. Upon returning home the jackal detected what seemed to be footprints at the mouth of the cave. Standing at a safe distance prepared for flight he shouted: "Oh cave, why do you not welcome me home? I cannot enter without your invitation." The less discerning lion responded: "Come in, oh jackal. This is your cave speaking. I await you!"

In the preceding chapters we have seen footprints of a beast but we have heard no warnings from within. The presence of serious difficulties, however, becomes evident when we inquire into events for which conventional explanation fails. Like the clever jackal we must contrive to let unseen difficulties announce their presence, and this is the objective of the concluding chapter.

VII

Conclusion: The Whole Awaits

In beholding the human body, the first thing that strikes us, is its LIFE. This, of course should be the first object of our inquiries,... for the end of all the studies of a physician is to preserve life; and this cannot be perfectly done, until we know in what it consists.

Benjamin Rush (1746-1813)

1. Medical Mysteries: The Events of the Whole

When we come to know 'the whole' the doors of science will be opened to an array of events heretofore banished as medical mysteries. These events, unexplainable by scientific laws in existence today have been considered not the norm, but exceptions to the rule. They have often been denied outright, or classified as medical curiosities with the implication that their significance is slight, and that they do not betray a tragic flaw in the fabric of contemporary medicine. As we shall see, however, they do portend the presence of an unseen difficulty − the dilemma of dualism.

These unexplained and unexplainable events, when fully understood, will elucidate the workings of the still unseen whole. That whole will not be a sum of parts, but a revolutionary new vision of a third dimension of reality. It will allow science to approach with confidence various enigmatic events including the placebo effect; the success of hypnosis in the cure of warts; the outcomes of 'self-regulation' therapies; influence of the 'will to live,' and the psychophysiologic states known as 'psychosomatic disorders.'

All of these events point to a question not yet asked and not yet answered by modern science, a question of incalculable significance for the future of medicine: To what extent are health and disease subject to voluntary control by individuals?

We are not referring here to well known preventive measures such as maintaining a balanced diet and an optimal body weight. We are not referring to avoidance of toxins, moderation in alcohol consumption, and refraining from substance abuse. We refer instead to an internal resource as yet untapped, a capacity native to the human organism.

That capacity, now veiled in mystery, accounts for the existence of the several enigmatic events to which we now turn.

a. The Placebo Effect

The so-called 'placebo effect' is incomprehensible apart from the whole. It was discovered more than once in the centuries following Descartes, but was summarily dismissed as incredible – too unlikely to warrant serious attention. It was a violation of the expectations of scientists and it was forbidden by existing scientific laws. In recent years it was rediscovered quite by accident and could not be dismissed because the results of rigorous scientific research repeatedly confirmed its reality.

Scientific experiments make use of "controls" or control groups, and without these the results of studies would be of little value. Suppose, for instance, that a researcher developed a vaccine for use in preventing a disease, and then administered the vaccine to everyone considered likely to contract that disease. Regardless of the outcome, even if no one did contract the disease, the researcher could not conclude that the results were due to the vaccine itself. Some other factor may have been responsible for the results because the study had no control group.

To test the vaccine, or any type of remedy, it is necessary to administer the medication to but a portion of the population and to observe *the difference* in results between experimental and control group outcomes. The control group is given a 'placebo;' an inert substance – a pill minus the active ingredient.

Before being put on the market, all drugs must be tested for effectiveness in this way. Common sense leads one to assume that an effective medication should show a dramatic difference between experimental and control group outcomes. After all, members of the control group 'only think' they are receiving a useful medication.

To the great embarrassment of 'hard science,' control group members show consistent signs of being affected by pills lacking active chemical ingredients. If a medication is for insomnia, for instance, controls expecting desired effects report greater ease in falling asleep. If the medication is designed to prevent drowsiness, having caffeine as the active ingredient, control group members given tablets with no caffeine, nevertheless report increased alertness and resistance to sleep. Such results are so reliable that a rule has been adopted. In order to be placed on the market, a medication must do better than a placebo; its effect must be more potent than a mere 'thought process.' It must bring about a change more dramatic than that brought about by the simple expectation that a change will occur.

To further the embarrassment of physical medicine it has been ascertained that an anticipated difference between experimental and control group outcomes is in many instances very difficult to obtain. The changes brought about by placebos are dramatic; not merely psychological, but physical or physiological as well. In other words, the control group's results are not 'all in their heads.' Placebos have induced observable changes in the condition of the stomach lining; in the symptoms of ulcers; in migraine and other headaches, and even in inhibiting the cough reflex. They have brought temporary relief from severe pain in wound patients in hospital beds, and in a study of vaccines for the common cold, a placebo group showed results equal to the experimental group in reducing the frequency of colds in the course of a year.

Though the recent discovery of this placebo effect was accidental, premodern theory predicted and explained the event, and insightful thinkers of the past few centuries have likewise observed with fascination this violation of the rules of modern medical science. Historic figures who have acknowledged the reality of the phenomenon and sought an explanation of its occurrence, have arrived independently at common explanatory principles. Three factors have been identified as involved in bringing about the results: the faculty of imagination, the hope of recovery, and the patient's confidence in both physician and remedy.

In the premodern era placebos outnumbered all other forms of therapy. This was due in large part to the medieval influence. The Dark Ages, many long centuries of neglect of science, extinguished the light of reason which formerly pertained to remedies. There were two types of medieval medicine. The more dominant type was 'faith healing.' Remedies consisted of chants, blessings and rituals, shrines and their whereabouts, exorcismic rights and the relics of Saints to be ingested or worn about the body. The healing power was not thought to

reside in the human constitution. It was explained by the direct intervention of God and the Saints. The cause of disease was likewise a
supernatural phenomenon – a punishment for sin, and the failure of
any remedy was due to the sufferer's lack of contrition or lack of faith.

In this same dark age, when physicians were no longer trained,
many varieties of quackery abounded. Remedies were as bizarre as it
is possible to imagine. Placebos ranged from the most precious and
valued substances: gold, precious gems and pearls, to the most vile and
revolting substances a patient could be induced to swallow: live
spiders, human feces, urine, menstrual blood and powdered bones.

With the decline of medievalism and the revival of ancient learning
came the need to substitute naturalistic for supernatural explanations of
successful outcomes of such extraordinary therapy. Pre-Cartesian
understanding of the whole furnished a powerful explanation of the
placebo effect.

As demonstrated in Chapter V, scholars of the fifteen and early
sixteen-hundreds made frequent references to the phenomenon
understood in classical antiquity by the penetrating minds of Plato and
his medical contemporaries. Plato discussed the use of "fine words" used
in his age as charms or spells to ward off illness. These words had
healing properties insofar as they created balance or harmony in the
soul. Medical opinion held that the most trusted physician heals best.
The effectiveness of any remedy was dependent upon the patient's level
of confidence. Galen stated that reports of success of religious charms
and chants were not the "fairy tales of old women." Their effects were
verifiable and should be taken advantage of by physicians.

Prior to the ascent of dualism, in the final century of holism's reign,
theory to explain the placebo effect was highly sophisticated. Because
imagination played a central role in the cause and cure of disease, any
method capable of inducing a change in this causal substrate could influence the disease process. Thus physicians wrote defenses of the use
of spells, chants, charms, magical rituals and so on.

These methods were effective only when the patient's imagination
was strongly influenced. When placebo-like remedies were employed,
both patient and physician were advised to "affect vehemently,
imagine, hope and believe strongly for that will be of great help." Only
a "strong belief" could change the pathological state of the sufferer, and
a strong belief could be imparted only when the patient placed "much
confidence in the physician."

In the age of holism, placebo therapy was but one means of utilizing the self-regulatory capacity inherent in human nature. No special rules were required to explain the phenomenon. Existing theory accommodated it with ease. In the post-Cartesian era, however, the opposite became the case. Existing theory forbade its occurrence, and placed the effect outside of the domain of physical science.

One century into the reign of dualism the scientific commission who discredited Mesmer claimed that as far as mesmerism's therapeutic successes were concerned: "the imagination does everything." This might appear to have been a vindication for pre-modern theory and a triumph for holism. But it was in fact the opposite. When modern scientists used the word *imagination,* it referred exclusively to a mental state. If imagination brought about a cure, the alleged disease was bound to have been an "imaginary ailment."

The placebos of the nineteenth century included metallic objects presumed to influence animal electricity or animal magnetism. When orthodox medicine protested use of these dubious methods, the claim was again made that imagination accounted for any and all therapeutic successes. The implication was that therapeutic success was in fact nonexistent, and that the effects were simply *not real.* Medicine condemned use of all remedies for which no physical basis of effectiveness could be found.

Despite this prevalent mode of thinking, a few eighteenth and nineteenth century physicians observed and insisted upon the reality of the effect. One of these was William Falconer who wrote in 1788 that numerous cures "have been performed by medicines of little, or even of no, medical efficacy whatever." These cures were said to depend upon the patient's imagination, and on "the opinion the patient entertained of their powers." Falconer offered as proof of the reality of the effect that the success of *any* cure depends upon the degree of the patient's confidence in the success of the remedy!

In the mid-eighteen hundreds, when Falconer's arguments had long since been forgotten, a physician named Daniel Tuke chanced upon a news' item which stimulated his curiosity. The article described a bloody and dramatic railway accident in which many persons were killed. Of the survivors, one emerged from the wreckage completely cured of a severe case of rheumatism. Tuke was struck by the insight that this medical curiosity might be of great significance for understanding disease and healing processes. He undertook a search of the literature for similar instances, and built a case for a causal role of mental influences on bodily functions.

His research led to the conclusion that the chief causal factor was imagination, and he perceived a relationship between the diverse events his search revealed. Imagination, insisted Dr. Tuke, allows inert substances to induce actual physical changes in the body. Why, he argued, should medicine not take advantage of this power? He described how bread crumbs could be encapsulated to resemble pills, and discussed the use of these pills for two types of disorders: nervous conditions and constipation.

As previously noted, the 'nervous' disorders of Tuke's era were the nineteenth century equivalent of our 'stress' disorders. The physician was correct in his supposition of the effectiveness of placebo therapy for these psychosomatic conditions. Bread crumb filled capsules taken from a box marked "purgatives" were used for the common complaint of constipation. Patients requiring a purgative were directed to take five of these capsules every quarter of an hour for a period of several hours' duration. Tuke described the remarkable effectiveness of this "most violent purgative."

Dr. Tuke's insights likewise failed to sway medical opinion, however, and were soon forgotten. Regardless of how powerful or forceful imagination was said to be, it remained a mental entity. As such it could not possibly exert any influence on the physical mechanisms governing bodily functions. Orthodox physicians were inclined to disregard the phenomenon rather than be compelled to confront its enigmatic basis.

With the modern proliferation of research documenting its reality came the virtual impossibility of denying or neglecting the placebo effect. Though dualism still obscures our understanding, modern discussion echoes voices from history. Contemporary opinion states that placebos depend for their force on the conviction of the patient that a given effect will result. This "conviction," wrote Drs. Rosenthal and Frank (1956), appears to be related to the patient's "confidence in his physician." These authors state, with Hippocrates, that the "authoritarian attitude of the physician" can lead to the necessary conviction. Hippocrates had recommended a great show of erudition on the part of physicians before prescribing remedies, with the objective of instilling confidence.

Modern explanation, however, remains mentalistic and therefore fragmentary. In the pre-dualistic era the placebo effect was explained by the same theory and by means of the same concepts which explained health and disease generally. Nothing new was required for effective analysis because the placebo effect was compatible with, rather than a violation of the rules of scientific medicine. It was but another manifestation of the same holistic processes governing other bodily events.

Similarly, when modern science achieves an understanding of the placebo effect it will at the same time achieve understanding of the remaining mysteries discussed in this chapter. They are alike manifestations of the workings of the still unseen whole. Placebo effects are but one manifestation of our largely unknown and unexploited power of self-regulation.

This self-regulatory capacity is exercised by each of us on a daily basis, but unwittingly, and frequently in a direction opposite that which might be salutary. Consider for instance the placebo effect in the context of adverse side effects. Scientists have reported cases of rashes and other adverse reactions to placebos indistinguishable from those found after taking real medications over a period of time. Self-regulation works as readily in a negative as in a positive direction. In ignorance of this we desire that physicians recount in detail the potential adverse side effects of prescribed medications. Being informed that nausea, for instance, is a possible side effect, our likelihood of being so affected increases dramatically. Our powers of self-regulation can be employed to preserve or to destroy health. The Age of Anxiety has inclined more toward the latter, albeit without any distinct awareness of what has been happening at the level of underlying causation.

As the placebo effect represents a self-regulation mechanism having a probable association with imagination, so it appears does the phenomenon known as hypnosis. As discussed in Chapter IV, hypnosis, was condemned by orthodox medicine as a fraud. It could not be adequately explained and therefore had to be denied. The concept of imagination figured into this controversy in two ways. By some it was used as an explanatory principle to account for the effects of hypnosis, just as it had been used to explain the placebo effect. By others, and indeed, during the same era, the concept of imagination was used to discredit advocates of hypnosis by refuting their claims. These opponents of mesmerism stated that the method was powerless because all of its effects could be explained by the operations of imagination, and therefore the somatic complaints of Mesmer's patients had no physical basis. In this context, one supporter of hypnosis avowed that he would sooner accept a "diabolic" explanation of his results than attribute them to the operation of imagination.

The conceptual link between the medical mysteries of placebos and hypnosis is reinforced by the concept of "suggestion." In the seventeen hundreds a critic of medicine wrote:

> The surest road to health, say what they will,
> Is never to suppose we shall be ill.
> Most of those evils we poor mortals know
> From doctors and *imagination* flow.

To "suppose we shall be ill" captures the meaning of expectation of outcome recognized as necessary to the placebo effect. The suggestions used in hypnosis tie in logically with this phenomenon.

Another critic of orthodox medicine, the author Romains, satirized medicine's "imaginary ailments." The central figure in the amusing story of *Knock, or the Triumph of Medicine* was an ingenious physician who took over the dwindling practice of another doctor. Observing that a living could scarcely be made on the existing practice, Dr. Knock used "suggestion" to increase his following. If a patient reported good health he probed until he found a minor complaint and then stimulated the imagination with vivid descriptions of what serious disorders that complaint might be symptomatic of Dr. Knock's method of suggestion was so effective that the health of the community deteriorated rapidly and a local hotel was converted into a hospital to accommodate the overflow. Critics accused Dr. Knock of treating "imaginary ailments" but the physician insisted that his diagnoses were never imaginary.

b. The Success of Hypnosis in the Cure of Warts

The placebo-effect, imagination, suggestion and hypnosis occupy the same conceptual category. They are events which disclose a capacity for self-regulation and they are events lacking fundamental explanation. The modern tendency has been toward independent psychological explanations for each of the mysterious events discussed here. Successful explanation, however, must ultimately identify a common law; a biotonic principle capable of unifying the more apparent than real diversity.

It was the mystery surrounding hypnosis, and not any lack of verifiability of its effects, which led to its condemnation by medical authorities. Even to this day its therapeutic potential has never been fully explored because an explanation satisfactory to all has not been achieved. Popular opinion presumes its effects, whatever these might be, to be minor, and thus not requiring a great deal of serious consideration.

Lewis Thomas, Chancellor of the Sloan-Kettering Cancer Center, had the insight to perceive instead the vast significance of one inexplicable outcome of hypnotherapy − the elimination of warts. When we achieve an understanding of how "warts can be ordered off the skin by hypnotic suggestion, wrote Dr. Thomas, we resolve "one of the great mystifications of science. Best of all," he continued, we find out about "a kind of superintelligence that exists in each of us."

Skeptics prejudiced by dualism have often minimized the importance of effects of hypnosis and other self-regulation strategies by reducing all to placebo effects. Although this tactic sustains confidence that medical theory is not grossly inadequate, it adds nothing to our knowledge of the means by which hypnotherapy influences warts, since placebo effects likewise remain unexplained at the most fundamental level.

In a controlled study Dr. Surman and colleagues (1973) treated seventeen patients for common or plantar warts by means of hypnotherapy. These patients, some with serious, long standing wart problems, were told to refrain from use of any home remedies. They were further informed that "the likelihood of cure with hypnosis" was as yet "highly uncertain." Though this caution might negate the placebo effect which relates to certainty and confidence in outcome, the results were highly impressive. More than half of the patients showed improvement, and several showed a complete disappearance of all warts within the three months of therapy, a finding which spontaneous disappearance could by no means explain.

Warts are caused by a viral agent. Crossing the gulf between a psychological "suggestion" and a pathogen defined as "a particle of nucleic acid enclosed in a protein," is an impossible objective for medical theory as it exists today. For this reason insurance companies typically refuse coverage for this type of therapy, even though for some individuals it appears to be *the only* effective method for treatment of warts.

c. The Self-regulation Therapies

Autogenic Training and Biofeedback

The emerging field of self-regulation is not represented by hypnosis or placebo use, but by a class of innovative methods looked upon with considerable suspicion by orthodox practitioners. These methods include autogenic training, biofeedback, progressive relaxation, a variety of meditative exercises and guided imagery.

Autogenic training emerged in Europe in the early years of this century for treatment of psychosomatic disorders. Its developer, J. H. Schultz, had observed the feelings reported by deeply relaxed, hypnotized patients. These, he noted, described the very states of body propitious to relief of various symptoms. Autogenic, or 'self-produced' bodily changes, are brought about by focusing attention on key phrases, such as "My arms and legs are heavy and warm." The majority of patients trained in this method over a period of months show substantial benefit. Concentration on the "autogenic phrases" brings certain involuntary functions under voluntary control. Medical theory has not been able to accommodate this apparent contradiction, though the method has found more favor abroad than in the United States.

Self-regulation was the rule rather than the exception in premodern medicine and it continues to thrive in countries less modernized or Westernized than our own. In India, for instance, training in yoga is commonplace and yogis perform feats of voluntary control of biologic mechanisms which have staggered the Western imagination.

The "yogic feats," as they have come to be called, involve self-regulation of processes to which the Cartesian mind, by definition, has no access. How has Western science interpreted these events? There have been two general means of coping with research findings confirming the reality of these counter-instances to theory. Some research has been discredited. Other findings have been forced into the established theoretical framework, although with an uncomfortable fit, as discussed in Chapter IV.

The Western approach, founded upon dualism, has been unable to evolve sound explanatory constructs for the yogic feats. As a consequence modern medicine has been unable to derive benefits from knowledge of their existence. Even in India, scientific medicine has not borrowed from traditional medicine. The two approaches share no common assumptions regarding the nature of the organism. They coexist rather peacefully in India however, and a trained physician will occasionally refer a patient to a practitioner of traditional healing strategies.

But in the U.S. we have known only physical medicine, and self-regulation methods remain shrouded in mystery from the orthodox perspective. Having offered self-regulation training for stress management over several years, I have observed that two segments of the physician population show receptiveness to these innovations. The first group is represented by youthful practitioners who have been educated in the effectiveness of these methods in updated medical curricula.

A second type of physician likely to be receptive is the very mature, experienced doctor for whom time and wisdom have been educators. This seasoned practitioner has come to know that illness is of another order of complexity than physical medicine specifies. Daily contact with patients over many years may bring insight into the self-destructive character of illness. From this it might be ascertained that self-regulation could through some method be made to operate in the reverse direction.

The causal basis of self-regulation effects, however, remains inexplicable. Neither mind nor body can claim responsibility for these effects which emerge instead from the still unknown and unnamed whole. To exemplify this problem of explanation consider the procedure known as biofeedback.

The word "biofeedback" conjures up images of a technologic wonder beyond the grasp of ordinary mortals. In fact, however, the procedure is of utmost simplicity. To explain its operation by analogy, suppose you wished to learn to hit the bull's-eye on a dart board, and a friend recommended that you practice wearing a blindfold. You would surely object saying; "If I can't see what I'm doing, how am I to learn?"

Now suppose the skill you wished to learn was lowering blood pressure. No matter how much confidence you had in your ability to perform this feat, you would refuse to practice in the absence of knowledge of results. Knowledge of results removes the blindfold and makes learning possible. That knowledge is called "feedback." It lets you see what you're doing.

Feedback from the bio-system or body opens a new world of skill learning. Persons observing their internal bodily processes by means of electronic feedback instruments have learned to modify blood pressure, readjust the flow of blood to various parts of the body, reduce tension in painful, tight muscles, and so on. The more one practices, the more skillful one becomes, just as one's learning progresses in skills like dart throwing or piano playing.

Why then is biofeedback grouped here with medical mysteries like yogic feats and hypnosis-wart cures? The answer is dualism and the problem of causal explanation. At the outset it is apparent that biofeedback cannot be fully explained by means of mechanical or physical causation. Skill learning has no analogue in the material world, nor can we deny the roles of sentience or intelligence, and the organism's ability to sense and perceive.

Dualism assumes that if explanation is not possible in physical terms the explanation must be mental. Perhaps the conscious mind can assume the weight of causal responsibility here. If, indeed, biofeedback is an instance of 'mind control' then persons after training "know how" to lower blood pressure as they "know how" to read and write.

After centuries of indoctrination our inclination is to attribute unlimited authority to the thinking thing; the wellspring of reason and will. But when we look to mind or thought processes for an explanation of control of blood pressure (or of other biofeedback trained skills), we find mind as helpless as a babe. When asked "How do you do that?," the person trained in blood pressure control is very likely to respond "I don't know." The glorified mind of tradition, the intellect presumed to govern human destiny, the conscious ego, self or I, has utterly no claim to control of this skill, and no insight into how it is effected. No strategy, no design, no plan, in short no conscious thought process need be involved in acquiring such control skills.

For persons skilled in controlling autonomic functions the Cartesian mind cannot lay claim to control powers which transcend insight, rationality and the "will" itself. Nor can material conditions offer explanation above and beyond description of underlying physiologic mechanisms. Some unknown third factor is at the basis of this phenomenon.

The mystery of biofeedback is not an oddity, however. Its mode of operation is a prototype of organismic functions incomprehensible apart from the whole. We accept without question that all voluntary movements of the body are controlled by the mind. Suppose, however, that someone approached you saying: "I cannot make a fist. How do you make a fist?" Your immediate impulse might be to demonstrate the act of fist making. But suppose the inquirer responds "I know what a fist looks like, but *how* do you make a fist?"

You are now in the clutches of the dualism dilemma which holds at bay effective concepts of causation. Biofeedback, hypnotherapy and placebo therapy do not submit to causal explanation in the mind-body framework. Some unknown third factor is necessary on logical grounds.

If you are a scientist you will describe fist making as electrochemical impulses conducted by synaptic transmission from brain to hand. You may go further perhaps to describe the physiologic basis of muscle contraction and to detail the activities of ion transport and cellular metabolism. The more precision you achieve in this analysis, the further you digress from the question which prompted it. It becomes clear that you are no longer addressing the question of how one makes a fist.

If your inclination is towards engineering you might make use of a model as Descartes did in the sixteen hundreds. Technology has come far in three centuries, however, and pumps and pipes are unlikely to impress your listener. You may command more attention with a computer model describing fist making by means of another language, and diagramming the process with flow charts. However sophisticated this analysis your questioner is no closer to a solution to the problem: "How do you make a fist?"

Physical or mechanical explanation, occupying one horn of the dilemma, fails to furnish a satisfactory answer. Mental causation of a physical mechanism, without the power of God uniting the two, likewise fails. If you resort to the unconscious mind as controller you are no longer talking about the mind as defined by tradition. The essence of the Cartesian mind "consists entirely in thinking." If some unconscious force or power is accountable for fist making, an unknown is brought into play. We thus arrive again at the same point — the necessity for a biotonic solution and the need to come to terms with the still unknown dimension of human nature.

Meditative Techniques

If biofeedback's effects appear somewhat mysterious, the effects of meditative techniques are orders of magnitude more so. Though autogenic training and biofeedback are grouped as instances of acquired conscious control of bodily functions, the effects of meditation resist even this loose and general classification.

The objective of meditation for self-regulation is not to "harness up" conscious powers. It is not to establish the dominion of mind, but to *silence* the mind itself. The meaning of this Eastern tradition is captured in the phrase "Thought is the disease of the Western mind." The objective of meditative exercises is not to train, but to obliterate the discursive thinking commonly referred to as mind.

Herbert Benson, a physician on Harvard's medical faculty, was courageous enough to acknowledge and to pursue the effects of meditation, particularly regarding his special interests, hypertension and heart disease. His popular volume titled *The Relaxation Response* (1975) was an attempt to demystify meditation and make its benefits more accessible to Westerners. It summarized some of the many research findings confirming the reliable bodily effects of meditation.

The general outcome of meditation represents a return to physiologic equilibrium or homeostasis, and makes one mindful of the premodern medical prescription of tranquility or quiescence. Bodily changes recorded include normalization of blood sugar and cholesterol levels, alteration in brain wave patterns, reduction in muscle tension levels, reduction of metabolic rate, reduced cardiac output, and numerous other bodily changes. These outcomes appear to reverse the stress process, and they occur in the absence of dangerous side effects.

If a drug were discovered which could safely accomplish all of this it would surely have swept the country. But meditation resists explanation and frightens most standard practitioners from its serious consideration, despite repeated confirmations of dramatically beneficial effects in research laboratories.

Meditative techniques typically involve the occupation of attention by continuous repetition of a word or phrase. This focus point for mind is meaningless and emotionally neutral. It may be a word from the ancient Indian language Sanskrit — a 'mantra' such as "Om," or it could be the word "one" used by Dr. Benson. It is designed to provoke no questions, no associations and to be neither good nor bad. It appears to act by monopolizing the mental apparatus and thereby preventing the occurrence of the usual stress ladened internal dialogue.

Talking to one's self from the moment of awakening to the twilight of consciousness preceding sleep is accepted as perfectly normal, but in all likelihood it is not beneficial to health. Typical discourse includes no small element of 'stewing:' "Just what did he mean by that remark? If he ever says anything like that to me again I'll". . . etc. The internal dialogue is more likely to place us in the unknown future than in present reality. We may worry our way through daily activities paying interest in advance on debts not yet due. Quieting this storm in the mind by means of meditative techniques could presumably reduce the activation and arousal levels with which the mental storm correlates. Yet the notion of mind as enemy rather than ally goes against the grain of Western tradition.

Our confidence in the powers of will and reason contradicts the facts of meditation outcomes. Instead of establishing 'conscious control,' meditation aims at *eliminating* it. The Zen doctrine of 'no mind' teaches the absurdity of the dualistic assumption that one 'has' a mind in the first place. Being "out of one's mind" signifies to us a pathologic state of insanity, but getting "out of one's mind" is the therapeutic objective of meditative exercises. For the Easterner, being *un*conscious of the feet means that the shoes fit confortably. Being at ease at the waist means *un*consciousness of the belt, and being unconscious of the very ease itself is what the true master of meditation seeks to accomplish.

Contrary to what our mentalistic tradition might assume, the "enlightenment" sought by serious meditators is not a realization of knowledge. To be fully enlightened is not to have acquired indubitable facts like those sought by Descartes. Enlightenment refers instead to a state in which one's being is purged of all delusion and duality. It is an achievement of unity, of being one with the universe, of transcending the mind-body dichotomy, not through rational thought but through direct experience. Neither mind nor body as traditionally construed can lay claim to authority as controller of this, or of other outcomes now known to derive from meditation.

The traditions of mentalism and mechanism give us no conceptual grip on these events. Were it not for an abundance of hard facts documented in research laboratories, we would gladly have dismissed the whole package as metaphysical, mystical gibberish. Nevertheless, our research results have not resolved the enigma of meditation, nor could such research possibly do so. As demonstrated in Chapter IV, discoveries in this nebulous, holistic category have been 'explained away.' The therapeutic potential of the method has not been exploited in the every day practice of healing. The philosophic implications of the transcendence of duality, the perception of unity, the Zen doctrine of "no mind," all of these have been completely overlooked. They point clearly to the unknown, to the third dimension to which Western science has not yet gained access – the biotonic phase of existence.

Progressive Relaxation and Guided Imagery

Like biofeedback, 'progressive relaxation' is a simple and effective method of learned control over a function normally beyond such control – muscle tension. Like biofeedback, it operates on a skill-learning principle. By gradually and systematically tensing and relaxing muscles, persons learn to distinguish between differences not normally perceived. They learn to discriminate between ongoing muscle states and thus to cultivate relaxed as opposed to tense muscles. Though one could hardly find this mysterious, progressive relaxation remains subject to a subtle and insidious prejudice. This method with other self-regulation strategies, is often thwarted by the tacit assumption that biological processes are simply not subject to an individual's control.

The prejudice of modern science is at times evinced in the assumption that though such control might be possible, it is probably slight and of little consequence. At times the prejudice is manifest in the trainee's querry: "What should I say to myself to facilitate the control mechanism?" If voluntary control is possible, it must surely be the mind's doing. The trainee is both disappointed and perplexed when told that the internal voice has no commanding role to play in self-regulation, unless the role involves silencing that voice.

Even after *successful completion* of training the prejudice may reappear. After all, isn't it more reasonable to assume that a physical cause accounted for physical effects? Could the changes not have been brought about by some modification in diet? Were they not attributable to some other factor such as a medication taken concurrently, or a change in job, home life or perhaps the weather? The trained individual may well remain as skeptical as the physician who doubts the efficacy of self-regulation. Human nature is not defined in such a way as to allow the reality of learned control of biologic mechanisms.

Several years ago another self-regulation strategy sparked a fiery and still smoldering controversy in the scientific community. It involved use of directed mental imagery as therapy for cancer. Its advocates were dealt with by orthodox medicine and public opinion in a way somewhat similar to that in which Mesmer was treated in the past century. That a mental process could influence a viral related process like tumor growth is every bit as unlikely as the cure of warts by hypnotic suggestion. Nay, unlikely is a poorly chosen word. Both events are *physically impossible.*

Nevertheless, a growing body of literature attests to the effectiveness of guided imagery in controlling various physiologic functions, and indeed in controlling the immune system related to the onset and development of cancer. Recent research has shown that a substantial percentage of patients diagnosed as having medically incurable cancer can improve, can survive beyond their original prognoses, and can in a few cases show complete tumor regression, with the addition of imagery and deep relaxation to standard therapy.

This imagery method, thought to be an innovation, is but another echo from premodern history. Like other self-regulation strategies it points to the still mysterious workings of the whole. Patients who succeed in the imagery − cancer treatment have several features in common. They view the imagery therapy as "strong or powerful," thus sustaining confidence in its effectiveness. Their directed images are of a certain kind. They imagine their cancer cells as weak, confused and easily destructible. The immune system is visualized as an army of white blood cells outnumbering cancer cells by a wide margin. These aggressive fighter cells destroy tumors, and their remains are imaged as passing out of the body in a natural way.

Some researchers have involved hypnosis in this treatment procedure, assuming that deep bodily relaxation and the hypnotic state are very similar. Clinical improvements in cancer patients have also been reported as results of self-regulation methods not employing imagery, such as intensive meditation and other relaxation procedures. Results have shown actual physical changes in the number and location of white blood cells, and in other physical properties of lymphocytes. There is sufficient scientific documentation of effectiveness of these techniques on the progression of cancer to warrant its immediate inclusion in therapeutic procedure.

Yet the problem of explanation has stifled that development. In 1980 *Psychology Today* magazine published an article titled "Images that Heal: A Doubtful Idea Whose Time Has Come." Opponents of the concept prefer not to allow patients with cancer this avenue of treatment. Logic and the laws of science tell us that such treatment cannot be effective. It is far easier to discredit research confirming the reality of the event than to live comfortably with such findings. After all, if these findings are reproducible and legitimate, orthodox medical theory is brought into question. No amount of research will allow a reconciliation of such differences and advocates of imagery therapy see the shadow of condemnation clearly. They are aware of its historic condemnation, and nothing has occurred in the past century to prevent history from repeating itself.

The 'Will to Live'

Almost two hundred years ago a pioneer in American medicine, Dr. Benjamin Rush, urged his colleagues to keep an open mind regarding influence of the 'will' in the healing process. He felt that the successes of mesmerism were attributable to the power of will, and he correctly perceived the potential significance of this possibility. Rush was confident that great benefit would derive from medical understanding of the workings of will.

The will is the operating principle of the Cartesian mind, and one might presume it even more intriguing to science than imagery or hypnosis. But will appears to have too heavy a shroud of mentalism to warrant its scientific consideration. Two hundred years since Rush's recommendation we remain completely in the dark, even with respect to the well known observation of the effects of "will to live" on life or death outcomes following severe trauma. The concept goes undefined in medical dictionaries and finds no explanation in medical texts.

The Psychosomatic Disorders

Medicine has divided all illness into two categories inclusive of each and every known form of pathology. There are diseases of the body, and a fundamentally different group of mental diseases. Let the reader try his hand at classifying a few. To which category does dermatitis belong — mental or physical?

A skin condition with visible tissue damage is obviously a "physical" condition. What if the disturbance is restricted to but one part of the body, say, the left hand? Still physical. What if this skin disorder occurs in response to wearing a ring, such as a wedding ring? Ah ha! An allergy, and physical through and through. An allergy is medically defined as that which is produced by an allergen. The allergen in this instance might be the metallic substance of the ring. As proof of the physical nature of this disorder we need only instruct the patient to remove the ring and watch the skin return to its normal healthy condition.

This rapid healing confirms the supposition of a clear and easily understood case of physical illness. But what if we instruct the patient to remove the ring from the left hand where it has been worn, and to place it instead on the right. What must we conclude if the dermatitis *does not occur* on the right hand, no matter how long the ring is worn there? Holding fast to our physical classification we deduce that immunity has been built up over time.

Observing no reaction to the ring's presence on the right hand has not destroyed our confidence that physical reactions have physical causes. Now, however, suppose we instruct the individual to return the ring to its original position on the third finger of the left hand, and the skin disorder reappears. What we have here is a clear case of "ring finger dermatitis;" a disorder classified by modern medicine as "mental!" This disease is not related to the physical substance of which the ring is composed, but to the emotional meaning of the wedding ring. The disease speaks a language of its own in words we have yet to understand — it is the language of the whole.

Conditions known as 'hysterical' are every bit as enigmatic as those termed psychosomatic. Let us consider another disorder defying classification into mental or physical categories. A woman consults an obstetrician reporting a cessation of menstrual periods, morning sickness and showing a distension of the abdomen indicative of several months of pregnancy. In rare instances the obvious diagnosis is not the correct one. In pseudocyesis or "hysterical pregnancy" the body simulates many signs and symptoms of pregnancy without the anticipated physical trigger for inducing these effects. This condition, its dramatic bodily manifestations notwithstanding, is classified as a mental disorder, a variety of hysteria. The lesson of history notwithstanding, the condition is often referred to as "imaginary" pregnancy, and its imaginary symptoms are very real indeed.

Into what category would the reader place 'stroke?' This condition occurs when blood flow to portion of the brain is blocked causing brain tissue deprived of normal circulation to cease functioning. Stroke is categorized as a physical condition with a physical cause. Yet if we trace the causal mechanisms back in time we arrive at the fight or flight response described in Chapter II. As a protective measure the threatened organism prepared for combat is able to control excessive bleeding from wounds which may be inflicted. The blood coagulation factor is increased as part of the fight or flight defense. If the stress response persists, this increased likelihood of blood clotting can be hazardous, since that clotting can form the physical basis of a stroke. Thus the phenomenon can be understood in terms of physical mechanisms, but not *fully* understood, and perhaps not meaningfully understood from the standpoint of prevention.

These diseases, and the "stress" disorders discussed in Chapter II, are as old as humanity. All of the tools and methods of modern scientific research have been directed at them with intensity for many decades. Yet stress diseases are present in our society in near epidemic proportions, and statistics indicate that every individual will, on the average, succumb to one or more of these diseases in the course of a lifetime. Nevertheless, they must be grouped here with "medical mysteries." They are unquestionably holistic events and as such they are incomprehensible within the framework of modern science.

Their onset in association with stress has been documented from several perspectives. Regardless of how 'stress' is conceived the association emerges. When stress is defined as a psychological event, such as "anxiety," we find the linkage. Experiments designed to provoke anxiety show correlated bodily events productive of illness, like increases in blood pressure and elevations in muscle tension. When students told that their intelligence is being tested are given difficult mental arithmetic problems, their bodily responses are caricatures of symptoms of disease.

When stress is defined in terms of habits or behaviors the same outcomes are observable. Drs. Friedman and Rosenman, specialists in heart disease, looked to daily habits and behaviors for an answer and identified what they called the "Type A" behavior pattern. They described this pattern as the "hurry sickness," a battle against time, which takes its toll on the cardiovascular system leading ultimately to hypertension, coronary artery disease or heart attack.

Still other definitions of stress are found in the literature and again, all point to the same linkage with illness. Some researchers conceive stress in terms of life events over which persons have little or no control, such as the death of a spouse, a financial setback, a change of employment, a change of address, a traffic citation and a Christmas vacation. The more life changes one undergoes in a period of time, the higher the likelihood of a major change in health status.

Stress then is subject to numerous interpretations and scientists have felt free to define it in any way they please. The correlation between stress and illness emerges regardless of definition, and the association appears irrefutable. Yet despite the enlightenment, the field of medicine has not been revolutionized by these findings. Science continues to seek underlying mechanisms; physical explanations of events encompassed by the word stress which might then be construed as causes, allowing eventual dismissal of causally inept psychological constructs.

Stress is a physical concept, as shown in Chapter II, and as such promises medicine more than it has been able to deliver. If stress researchers are in fact dealing with psychological variables camouflaged so as not to resemble mental influences, the concept of stress will not take us to our destination. This difficulty is already evident in the literature. The most widely used medical text in the world, the *Merck Manual,* had this to say of stress in its 1982 edition. "In a great variety of disorders, psychological and social stresses are entwined." However, "cause and effect are difficult to disentangle" in investigating such associations, and the "mechanisms responsible for such symptoms are unclear although they are generally ascribed to tension (p. 1405)."

If "stress" has not solved the problem of causation, it is unlikely that "tension" will serve the purpose. Thus we find a troublesome ambiguity; an aura of mystery still surrounding the psychosomatic disorder. Dualism has been well camouflaged by "stress" and "tension" but the embarrassing secret cannot remain forever concealed. It will reappear at such time as the fundamental question is addressed. Exactly what is *psychosomatic* illness?

For accurate diagnosis physicians make use of diagnostic manuals which define for them exactly what constitutes a disease. These manuals have for three decades confirmed the reality of a class of disorders known as "psychosomatic." The joining of the word roots "psyche" and "soma," mind and body, pointed to a unique phenomenon − a physical disease with a psychological causal basis.

In 1980, the diagnostic manual published by the American Psychiatric Association *dropped its listing* of this classification of disease. In its place we find "physical conditions" which may be "affected," not caused, by psychological factors. What precisely is meant by "psychological factors?" This, the manual states, is very difficult to define. Dualism appears to have triumphed again, and logic has ruled the day at the expense of progress.

The stress concept is also in immediate peril of falling before the guns of logical reasoning. It can survive only with the realization that it represents not mental and physical causes but something totally new. It cannot be made to harmonize with existing theory in physical medicine. It is not compatible with mechanistic concepts of disease causation. Stress and psychosomatic illnesses remain mysteries to be explained, and that explanation will not come in the form of 'special rules' to account for unusual events.

2. The Necessity for a Revolution in Medicine

In the history of science we find many cases of atypical events which failed to fit into established conceptual models of nature. Many centuries ago the science of astronomy made use of a model which worked well in predicting the changing positions of the planets and stars. With the passage of time, however, astronomers accumulated numerous observations which did not conform to this model. The difficulty did not lead these scientists to forsake the model, but rather to modify it; to devise special rules for addition to the existing framework.

Though the system of prediction became increasingly overburdened and confused, it was not forsaken until a new model became available. Thus occurred the Copernican revolution which substituted a new model for astronomy involving the earth's rotation around the sun.

The ingenious work of Thomas S. Kuhn has taught us that this historic event is a prototype of how science advances. Discovery of events not predicted by existing models does not lead scientists to forsake their theoretical views of nature. A new model, such as the Copernican system, must be available before a revolution in science occurs. The medical mysteries discussed here, the hypnosis – wart cure; the influence of mental imagery on white blood cells and the immune response, etc.; these could be multiplied one-hundred fold without furthering the progress of science.

Science progresses only when discoveries like these point to the fact that existing theory *is wrong*. In Chapter IV we observed how discoveries of events not predicted by theory have been explained away or explicitly denied. Mental healing was a form of quackery and its method a "fraud" and a "hoax." Yogic feats were part trickery and part misrepresentation, being in reality cases of voluntary control of *voluntary* functions. Mesmer was an audacious and successful swindler whose patients had "imaginary" ailments. Psychosomatic conditions were found in the final analysis to be "physical" conditions. Hypnotically induced lesions of the skin were nothing more than "medical curiosities."

All of these phenomena have been interpreted so as to shelter and preserve the existing medical model. Yet to unbiased, unprejudiced observers they all point in the same direction. They point to a gaping deficiency in the existing model; to an unknown factor necessary for successful explanation. They point directly to the whole of human nature; an out and out violation of the dualistic model upon which scientific medicine rests. If the stress diseases and the remaining medical mysteries discussed here are neither mental events nor physical events, what are they?

The placebo effect, biofeedback, meditation outcomes, guided imagery and so on, embody our capacity for self-regulation. The stress diseases embody the same process gone awry. Hereditary predispositions play a role, specific life circumstances and other factors shape the process, but at base we have a permutation of the whole. The organism under its own influence creates health or disease as part of an autonomous life process.

The human faculties have been conceived as mental since the advent of Cartesianism. Our mental powers have included thinking, feeling, willing, imagining, remembering and so on. The bodily or physicochemical mechanisms of the organism included digestion, reproduction, growth, movement and so on. The total picture made no provision for 'healthing' or 'diseasing' as human faculties or powers.

For any disorder it is possible to present an elaborate and precise description of causation in physical terms. In ring finger dermatitis, for instance, science has still to discover some of the intricacies of its physico-chemical basis. Yet whole volumes could be devoted to its psychological basis and unconscious causal mechanisms. The two types of analysis will never result in the same conclusions. They will never converge at the same point. They will forever concern parts which cannot be combined to form a whole. Neither part can account for the undeniable presence of self-regulatory capacities. The biotonic dimension must be called into play if holism is to acquire genuine meaning.

"Holism," as a sum of the parts, has found great vogue in our era and has led to improved general health. There is ever present a dawning of awareness that health transcends the condition of the physico-chemical substrate. Persons combine vitamin consumption with jogging and massage. They attempt to avoid fats, substance abuse and stress. Yet they have not seen their true potential which for the most part remains dormant. Our powers extend far beyond what can be gained through presently conceived correct habits and hygiene. How much further beyond remains to be decided.

Those who have pointed in the correct direction have been voices crying in the wilderness. In 1979 a book appeared titled *Wholistic Health*. Donald Tubesing, its author, portrays the current state of health care with vividness and accuracy. "Something is wrong," he argues, the health care system is based on a "technological imperative." The tendency in medicine is to do anything it is technologically possible to do. "No other culture, at no other time in history, has approached illness and its treatment in such a mechanical, scientific, piecemeal, and divided manner (p.29)."

Dr. Tubesing does not analyze the historic and philosophic roots of modern medicine's problems, but it is apparent that dualism forms those roots. "Wholism," Dr. Tubesing urges, is the solution, and the book abounds with valuable insights and practical recommendations for resolving present difficulties. Were its wisdom applied the savings in costs and suffering would become readily apparent. We would come to know the benefits of prevention and nonchemical modes of treatment. We would see, as Dr. Tubesing puts it, that we as individuals "create our own bodies, our own health (p.222)."

The positive potential of this whole-person approach stands in dramatic contrast to an ominous passage in the book's forward: "I have frequently been told that 99 percent of doctors would be unwilling to practice medicine in the wholistic mode (p.11)." Regrettably, this estimate is probably accurate. Dualism mandates the traditional approach and will continue to do so until holism is given meaning at the most fundamental level. A revolutionary reconceptualization of human

nature is required. The philosophical hard core of medical theory dictates medical practice, and its current structure fails to furnish logical
justification of holistic alternatives.

We have come again full circle to the philosophy upon which
medicine and the human sciences rest. We have found that it is not
enough to find fault with modern methods; it is not enough to provide
insightful alternatives for health care delivery. Neither will violations
of our expectations precipitate necessary changes. The counter-
instances to theory such as yogic feats and hypnotically induced lesions
of the skin, have not and will not revolutionize medicine. What we require
is the toppling of the conceptual structure and a reconstruction from the
bottom up.

When we reach our destination, "physical" disorders will appear exceptions to the rule. The counter-instances to present theory will be
models of normal functioning. The self-regulation procedures may
well become first choices as opposed to last resorts in healing
strategies. The current medical objective of prolonging life may be
dwarfed in importance by a new vision of the meaning of well-being.
We may come to conceive health not as the absence of physical
pathology, but as the positive fulfillment of human potential.

The Cartesian dichotomy has defined human nature in such a way
that our greatest resource, our capacity for mental and bodily self-
regulation, has gone unrecognized. The facts of history delineated in
preceding chapters are incontrovertible. Yet one might still wonder
how a philosophy could conceivably determine so fundamental a
dimension of Western civilization. Is not philosophy an obscure subject
matter of concern to only a few scholars? How could a philosopher
writing in the sixteen hundreds have sealed our fates and defined for
each of us exactly what we are?

In the present day philosophy *is* for the most part an obscure subject
matter and its practical relevance to individuals is limited. Few
philosophers write for the lay audience. Over the centuries the writings
of these scholars have become increasingly difficult to comprehend,
and philosophers have progressively sequestered themselves in the
ivory towers of academia.

In Descartes' time, however, philosophers wrote best-sellers. In that
era of uncertainty people read philosophic works with the objective of
self-definition, especially with regard to questions of the soul, its
essence and its destination. Descartes told his audience what they

wanted to hear, and he told it with conviction and absolute confidence. He wrote in a captivating first person style, easily comprehended, and difficult to dispute without violating the tenets of received religion.

Over time Descartes' words were transformed from propositions to axioms − truths held beyond question. The mind-body problem, though universally recognized as a necessary implication of Cartesianism, became a 'fact of life;' an unwelcome but gratuitous part of the package.

Losing sight of its philosophic origins, science dismissed the mind-body problem as a philosophic or semantic difficulty. If a problem existed it was of no concern to scientists. Thus the problem became invisible, and with it disappeared our vision of the whole and our potential for self-regulation.

According to the Cartesian definition the human mind is entirely preternatural, having no natural explanation or cause. This mind is made for the world beyond, a supernatural entity definable only in terms of the opposites of the natural world. Body, as part of the universal mechanism, partakes directly of no aspect of this mind's domain.

As the modern scientific world-view took form, the theologic and mystical aspects of Cartesianism became less conspicuous. As a subject of natural science, the body would now be approached like the atom or the reaches of space with the objective of technologic conquest. The human intellect was set in opposition to humanity's physical nature, and mind and body as antagonists were thus estranged from one another, the occupants of disparate worlds.

So profound has been the influence of this metaphysic that a reference to "I," the ego or the self, is typically a reference to the Cartesian mind. This isolated entity dwells passively in the physical frame until destroyed by the corruption of matter composing that frame. The intellect, presumed to be the essence of what makes us human, is estranged from the rest of creation, and human beings are helpless captives of the body's governing principle - physico-chemical mechanism. According to Cartesianism we are strangers here, irrevocably disunited from body and material universe.

As a principle of theology the metaphysic disuniting mind and matter has served its purpose admirably. Theology is the justification, the true source and the rightful place of mind as immortal spirit. The dualistic metaphysic has likewise served the physical sciences, furthering progress by virtue of its reductionistic simplification of matter. But that which the dichotomy omits now cries out for explanation. The third dimension of existence, that which is neither immaterial mind nor inanimate matter, the biotonic dimension, completes the world-picture.

Within this realm of being lies vast potential for explanation. It permits a redefinition of human nature wherein self-regulation may be considered the norm. It allows us to conceive the organism in such a way that mind-body interaction is not necessary for the performance of control of biologic processes. In doing so it dispells the mystery surrounding the 'medical curiosities' discussed herein, and removes the prejudice attached for three centuries to non-physico-chemically based healing strategies.

Both mind and matter as defined by tradition are impotent in the realm of self-regulation. Since a vast body of literature documents the reality of self-regulatory performances we must empower the organism with this innate capacity. The potential benefits for health maintenance are vast since the new perspective has implications for as much as seventy percent of illness. The stress disorders may be reconceived in such a way that hopeful prospects for remediation replace grim outlooks prevalent today. When the directive "Learn to control it" replaces recommendations to "Learn to live with it," we rise to meet a challenge envisioned in antiquity. We see again the wisdom in the ancient therapeutic recommendation: "Bring under submission to thyself all that is thine own."

Physical medicine's failure with stress diseases points to the fact that body is not a simple physico-chemical mechanism. Certain disease states refuse to be conquered by an arsenal of technologic wonders and will not submit to conceptual analysis in mechanistic terms. Rather, the disease process is somehow 'intelligent' and speaks a language foreign to the ear of contemporary physical science. Biologic processes manifest an element of meaning which mechanistic models can never capture.

There is indeed a wisdom, not of body but of the whole which we observe in symptom formation, and this wisdom remains to be defined and employed to positive advantage. Medical science will be free to explore this avenue only when liberated from the dilemma posed by dualism, and at such time as this liberation is accomplished, the full meaning of "integrity" will be restored to the human organism.

References

Asterita, M. F. *The Physiology of Stress*, New York: Human Sciences Press, 1984.

Benson, H. *The Relaxation Response*, New York: William Morrow, 1975.

Burton, R. *The Anatomy of Melancholy* (1621), New York: Farrar and Rinehart, 1927.

Friedman, M. and Rosenman, R. *Type A Behavior and Your Heart*, New York: Fawcett Crest, 1974.

Heidbreder, E. *Seven Psychologies*, New York: Appleton-Century-Crofts, 1961.

James, William *The Letters of William James*, (Henry James, editor) Volume II, Boston: Atlantic Monthly Press, 1920.

Kaslof, L. J. *Wholistic Dimensions in Healing*, New York: Doubleday, 1978.

Kuhn, T. S. *The Structure of Scientific Revolutions*, Chicago: University of Chicago Press, 1962.

MacLeod, A. W., Wittkower, E. D., Margolin, S. G. Basic Concepts of Psychosomatic Medicine. In *Recent Developments in Psychosomatic Medicine*, E. D. Wittkower and R. A. Cleghorn (Eds.), London: Sir Isaac Pitman and Sons, 1954.

Pavlov, I. P. *Lectures on Conditioned Reflexes*, New York: International Publishers, 1928.

Penfield, W. The Electrode, the Brain and the Mind, *Z. Neurol. 201*, 297-309, 1972.

Rosenthal, D. and Frank J., Psychotherapy and the placebo effect, *Psychological Bulletin*, 1956, *53*, #4, 294-302.

Schrödinger, E. *What Is Life?* Cambridge: Cambridge University Press, 1945.

Sechenov, I. M. *Reflexes of the Brain*, Cambridge, Massachusetts: The M.I.T. Press, 1965.

Sheikh, A. A. (Ed.) *Imagination and Healing,* Farmingdale, New York: Baywood Publishing Company, 1984.

Surman, O., Gottlieb, S., Hackett, T., Silverberg, E. Hypnosis in the Treatment of Warts, *Archives in General Psychiatry,* 1973, reprinted in *Advances,* 1983, *1,* 18-26.

Szasz, T. S. *The Myth of Mental Illness,* New York: Paul B. Hoeber, Inc., 1961.

Tubesing, D. A. *Wholistic Health,* New York: Human Sciences Press, 1979.

Weimer, W. B. and Palermo, D. (Eds.) *Cognition and the Symbolic Processes* (2 Vols.), Hillsdale, N. J.: Erlbaum, 1982.

Wigner, E. P. *Symmetries and Reflections,* Bloomington: Indiana University Press, 1967.

.